Getting Ready for My X-Ray

An X-Ray Book for Kids

This book belongs to:

Written by Dr. Fei Zheng-Ward   Illustrated by Moch. Fajar Shobaru

Copyright © 2026 Fei Zheng-Ward

All rights reserved. Published by Fei Zheng-Ward, an imprint of FZWbooks. No part of this book may be copied, reproduced, recorded, transmitted, or stored by any means or in any form, electronic or mechanical, without obtaining prior written permission from the copyright owner.

Identifiers: ISBN 979-8-89318-138-8 (eBook)
ISBN 979-8-89318-139-5 (paperback)
ISBN 979-8-89318-140-1 (hardcover)

Have you ever taken a picture before? ____ YES   ____ NO

Have you ever wondered how doctors can see <u>under</u> your skin?

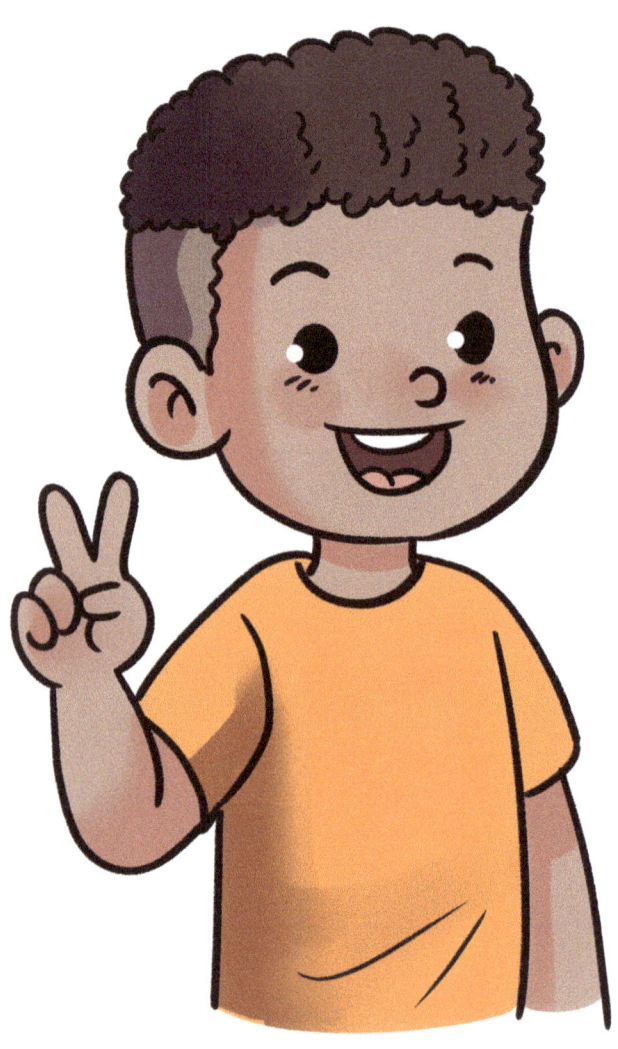
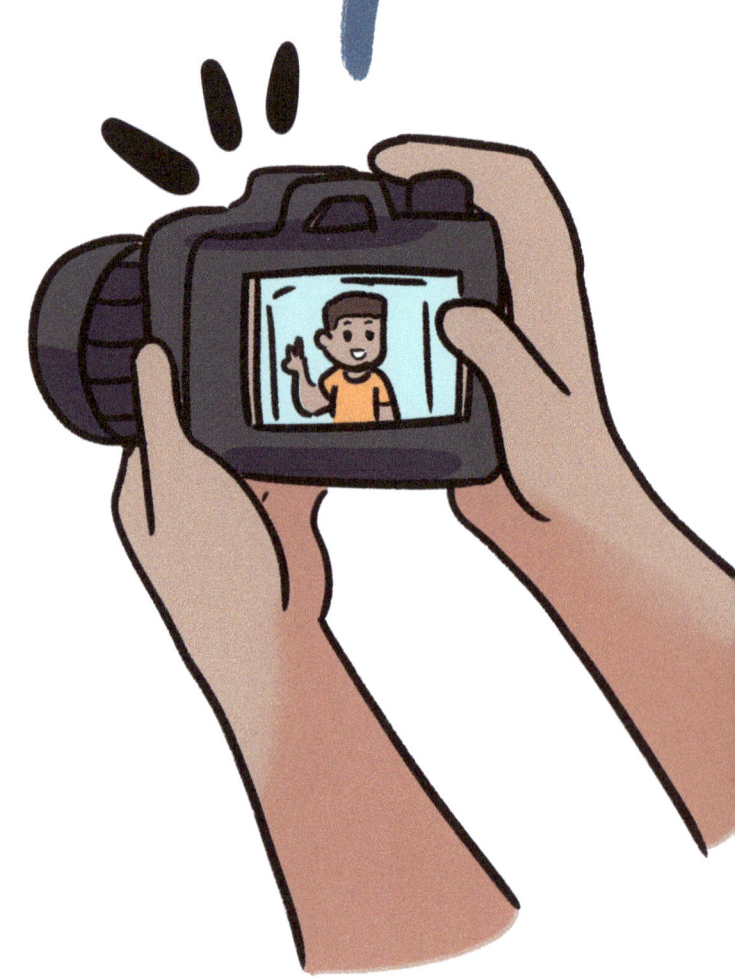

A special X-ray camera can do just that!

An X-ray is a special kind of picture that lets your doctor see inside your body.

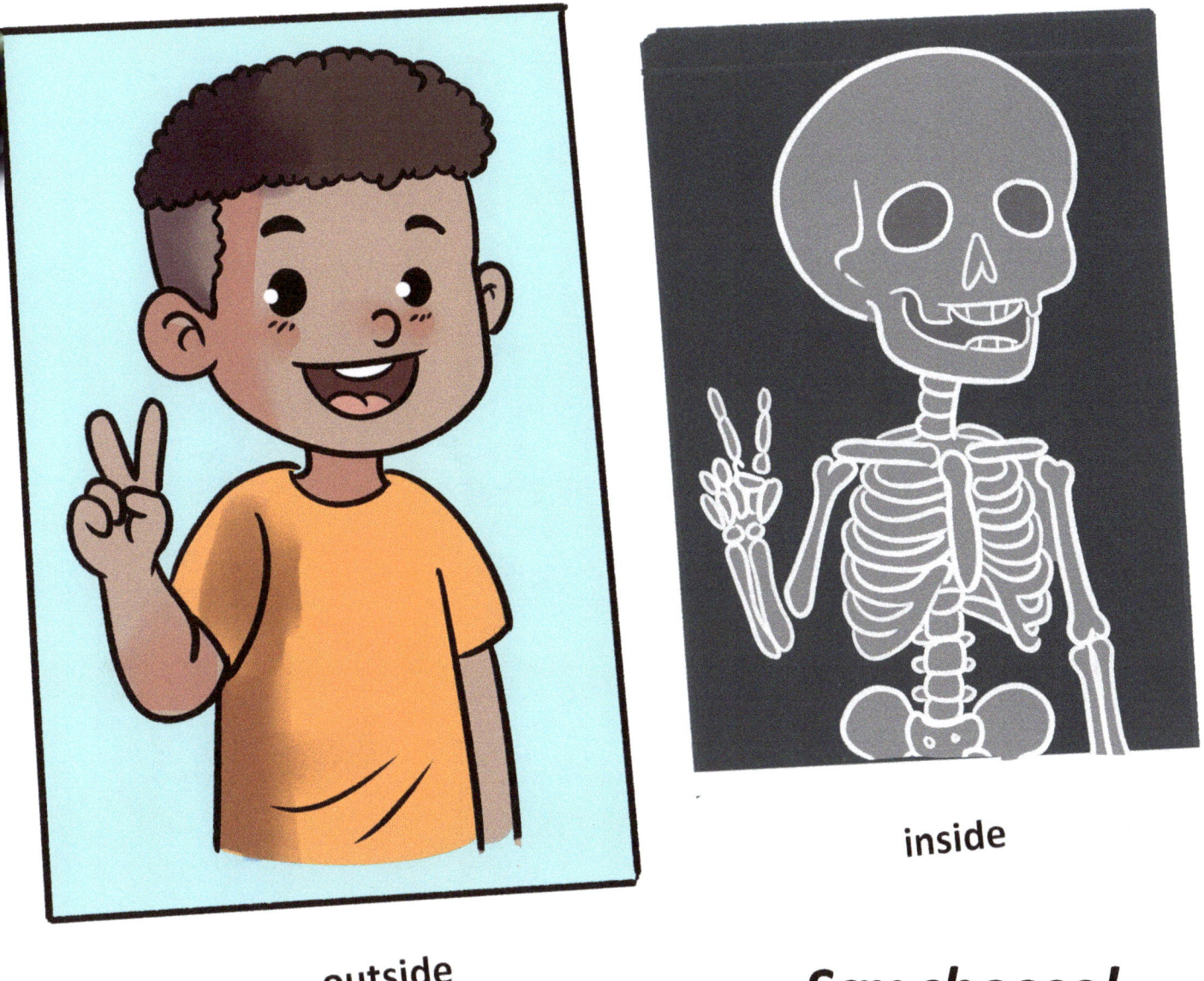

outside

inside

Say cheese!

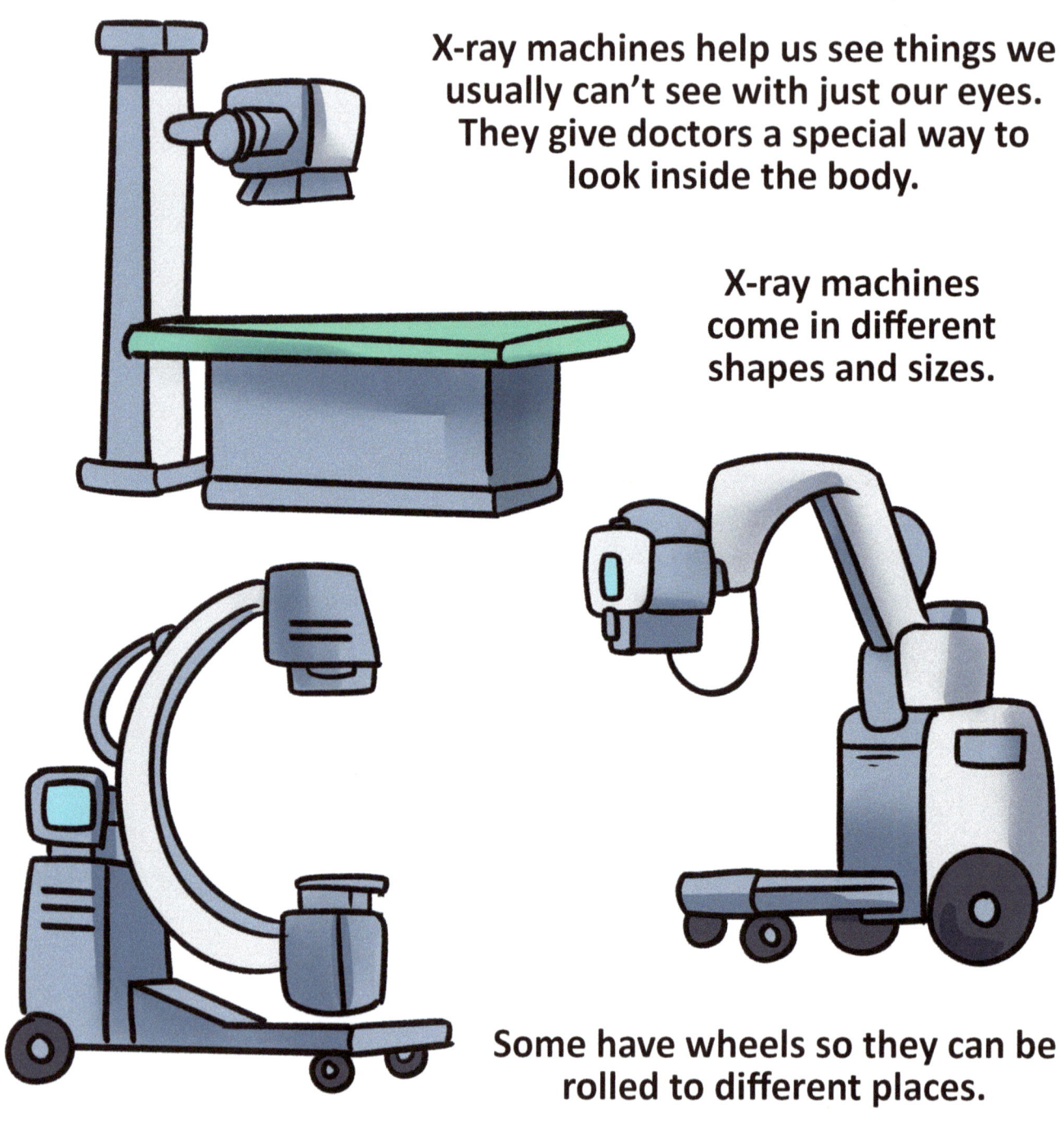

X-ray machines help us see things we usually can't see with just our eyes. They give doctors a special way to look inside the body.

X-ray machines come in different shapes and sizes.

Some have wheels so they can be rolled to different places.

Some are small and can be held with one hand.

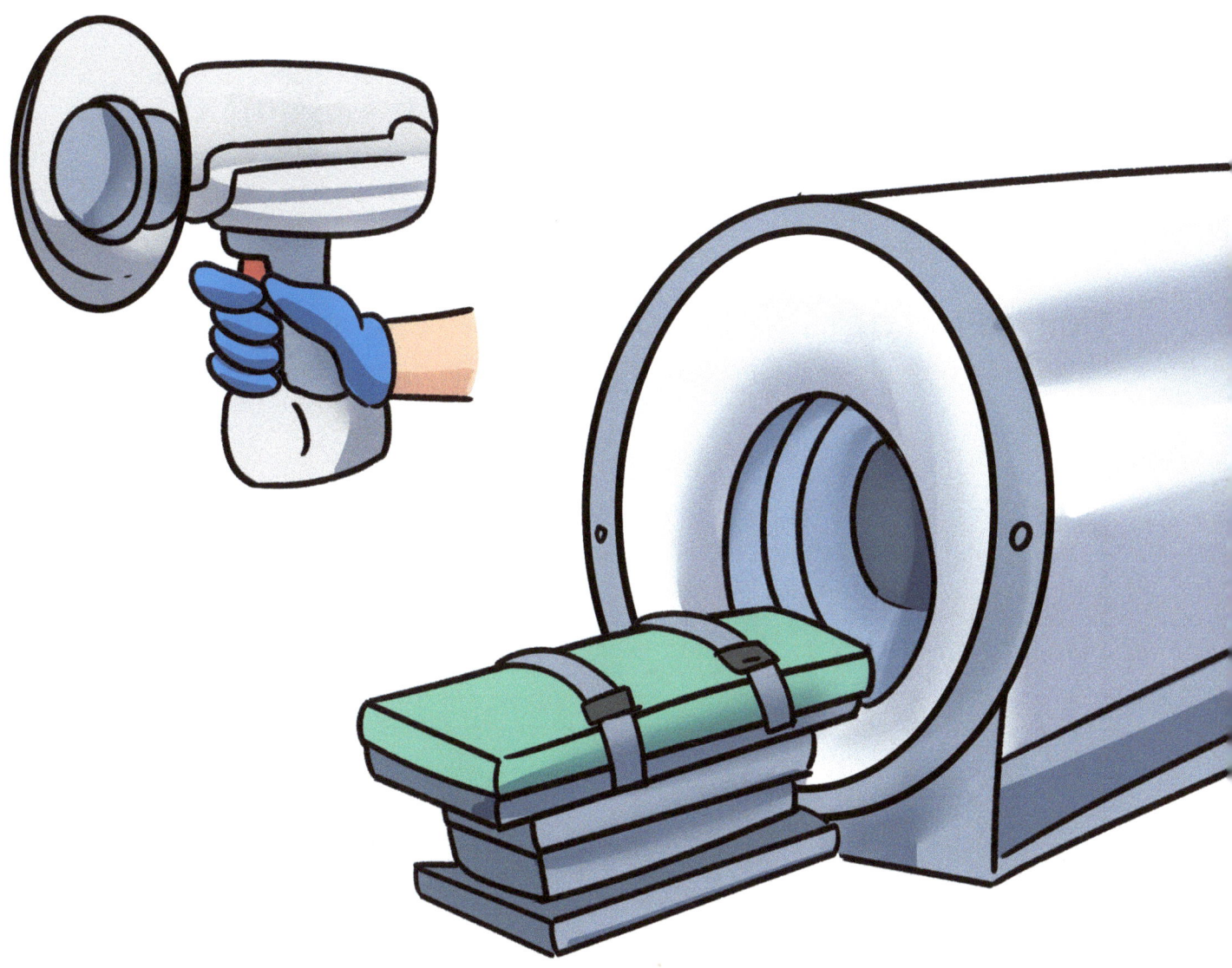

Some are so big that they fill almost the whole room!

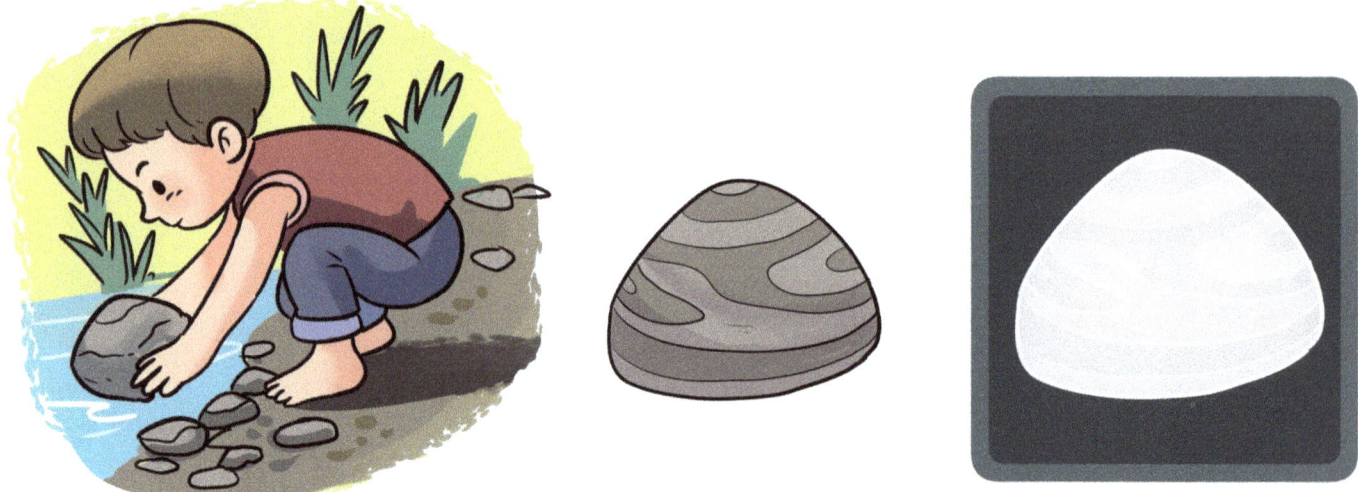

Things like **rocks and bones** are strong and tightly packed.
They show up on X-ray pictures as **white**.

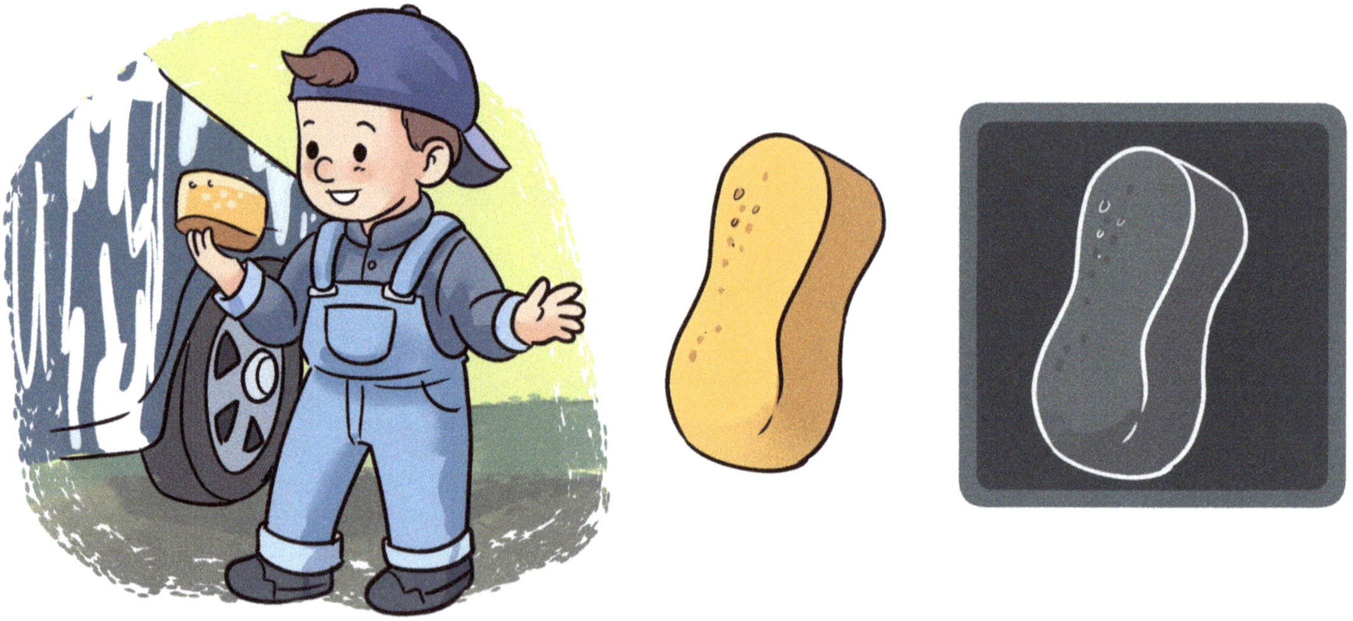

Things like **sponges and lungs** have lots of air inside.
They show up on X-ray pictures as **darker**.

Different parts of your body are made of different amounts of air, water, and bone— that's why they look different on X-ray pictures.

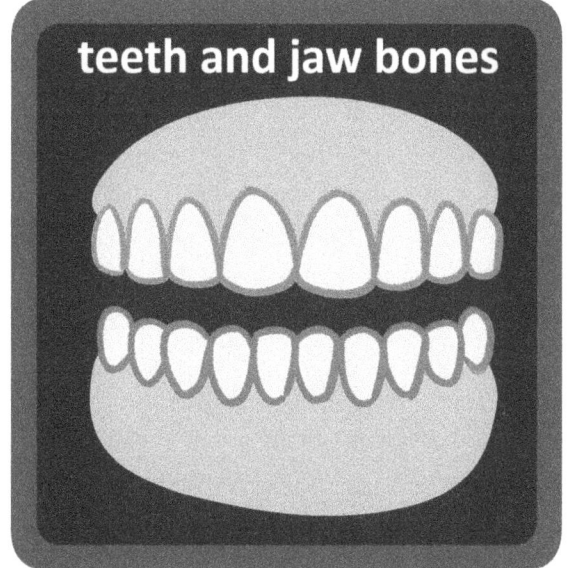

teeth and jaw bones

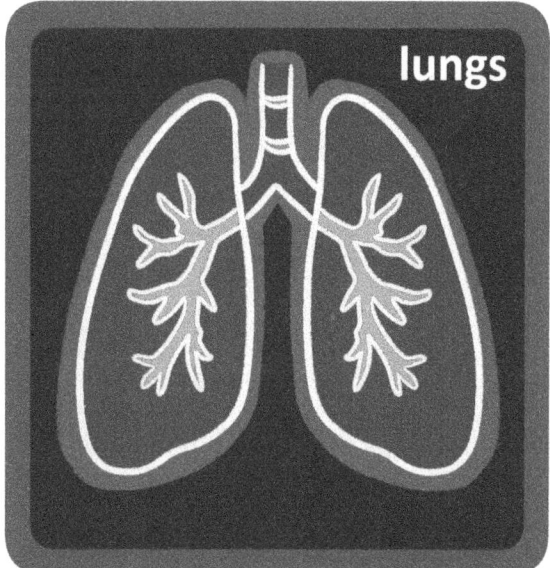

lungs

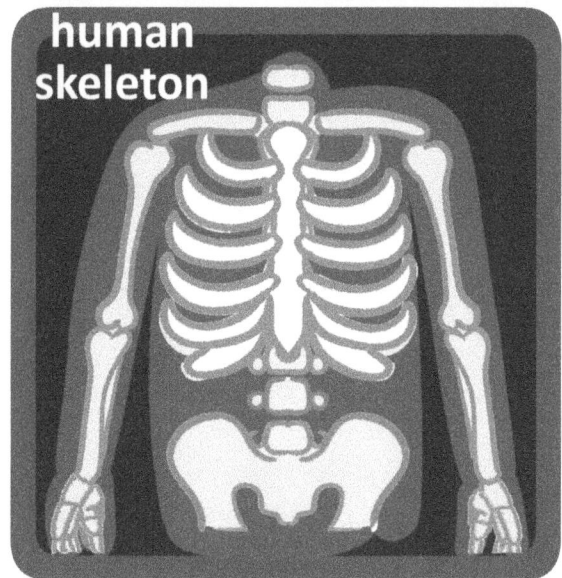

human skeleton

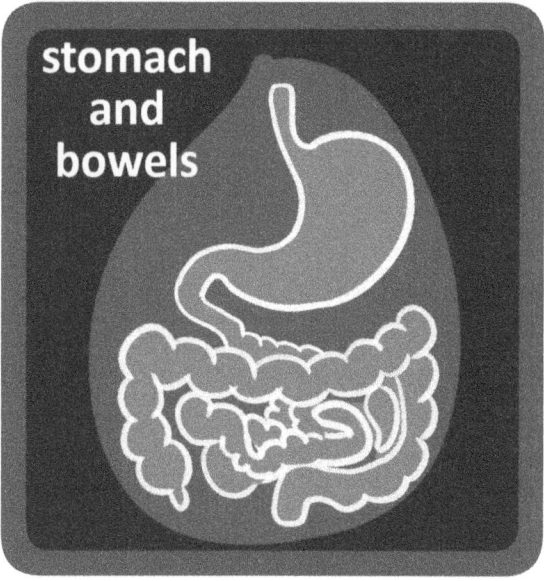

stomach and bowels

Have you ever had an X-ray before?

____ YES   ____ NO

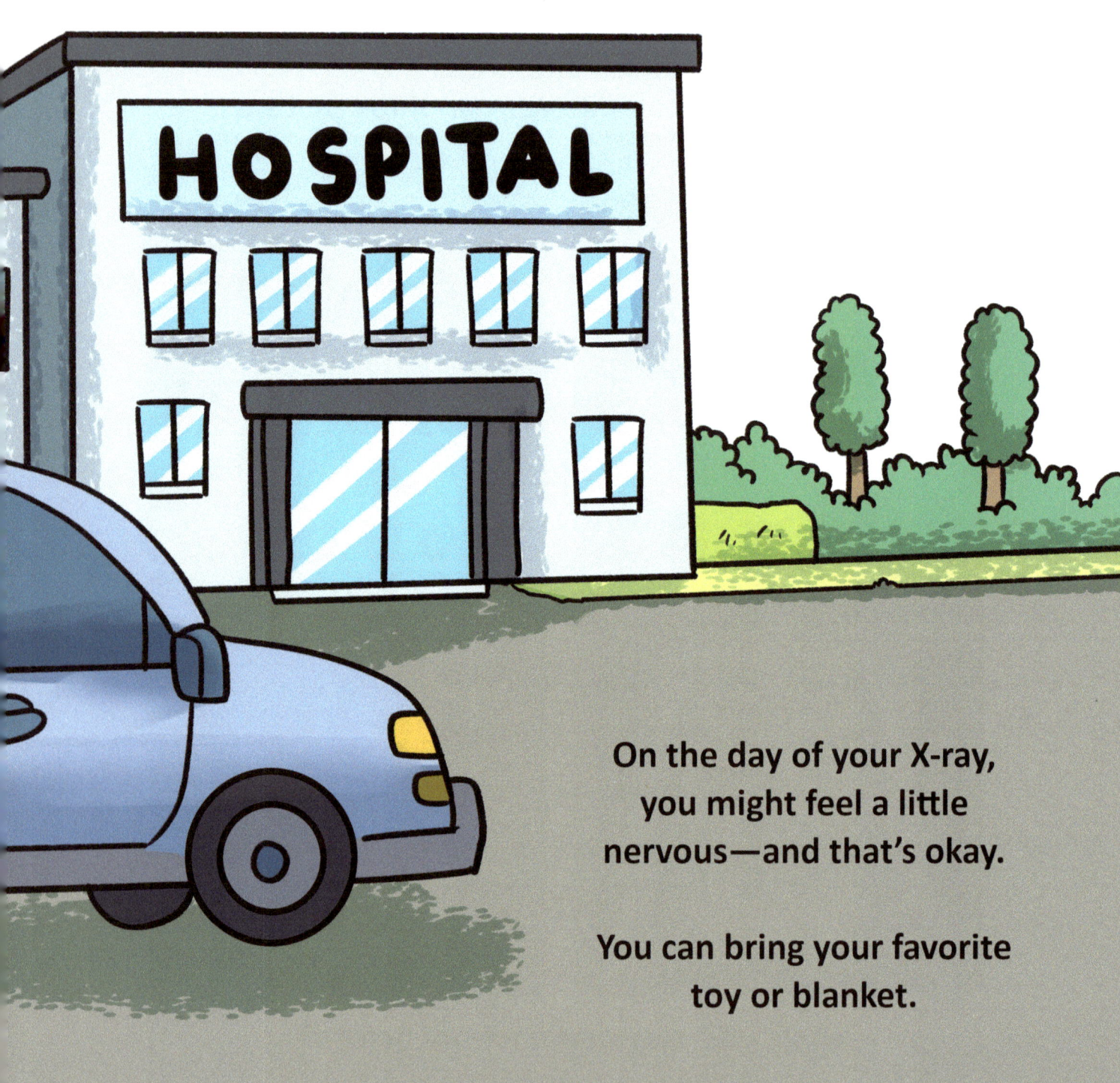

On the day of your X-ray, you might feel a little nervous—and that's okay.

You can bring your favorite toy or blanket.

What would you like to bring to your X-ray? Circle your answer.

Toy   Blanket

Other: _____

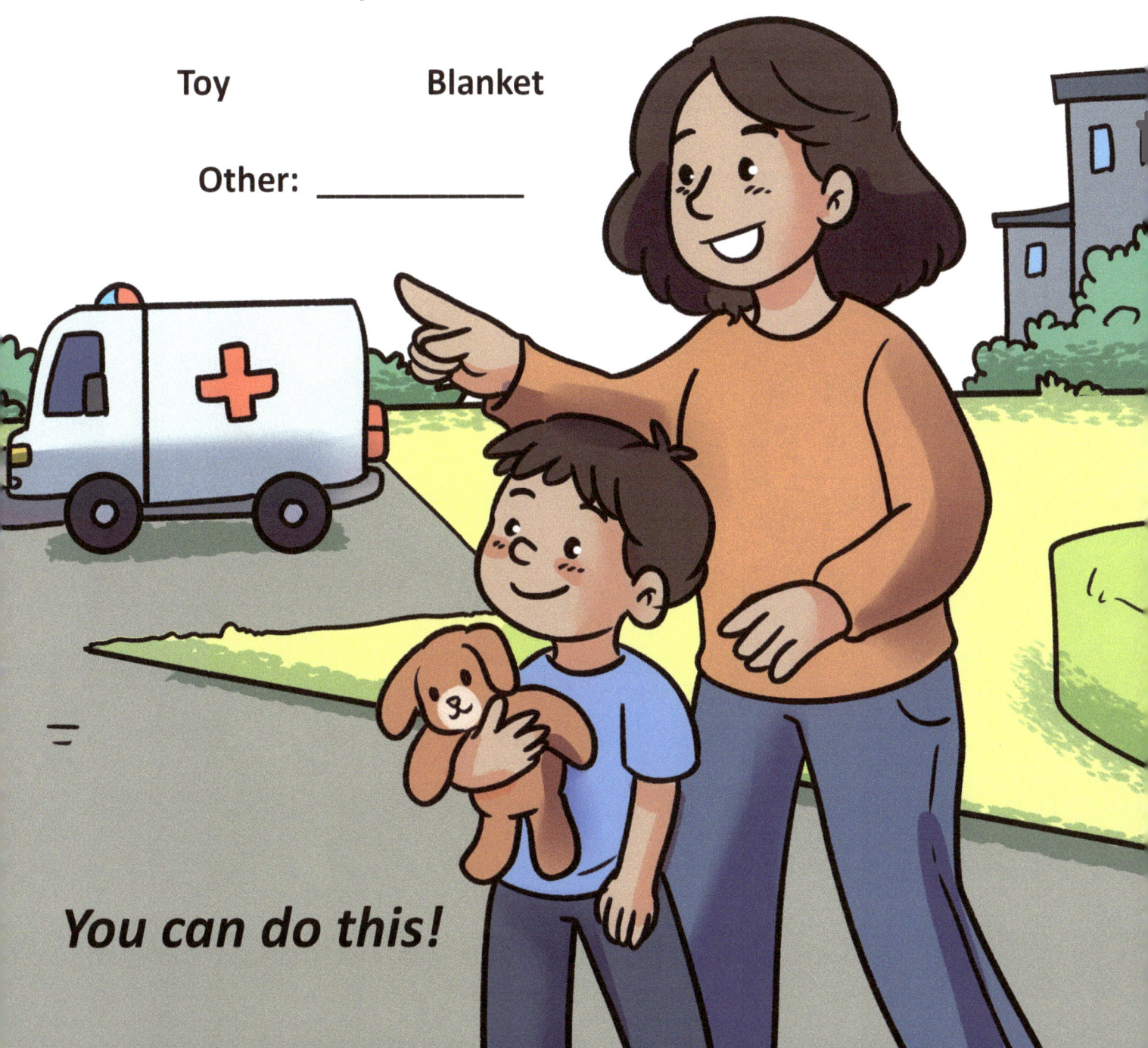

You can do this!

When you arrive, you'll check in and tell them your name and birthday.

They'll give you a special wristband so everyone knows who you are.

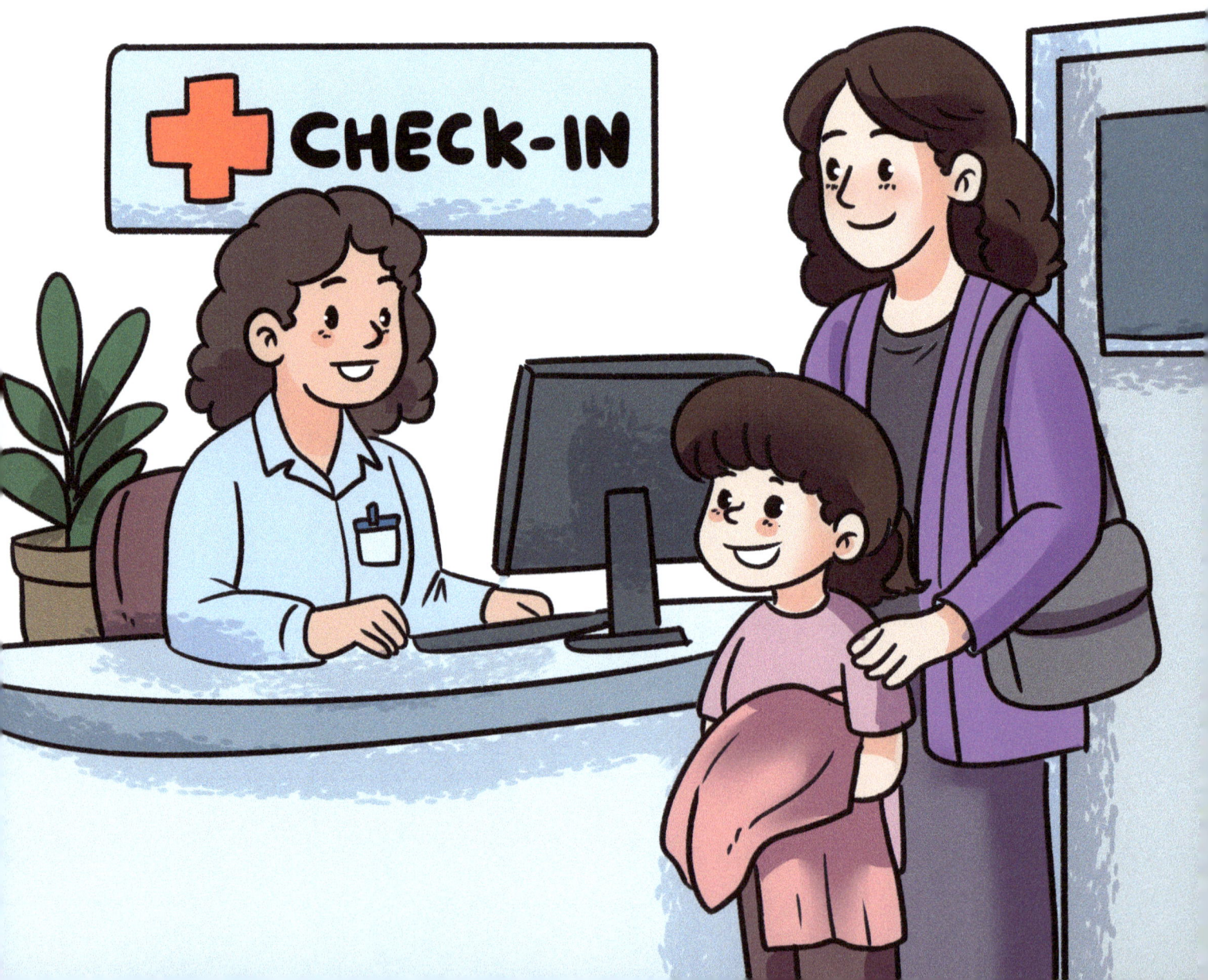

What color wristband will you get?
Circle the color of <u>your</u> wristband below.

Red   Green   Yellow   Blue   Pink   Orange

Purple   Black   White   Other: _____

After checking in, you and your parent or guardian will wait in the waiting room until it's your turn.

_____, you've got this!
(Write your name above)

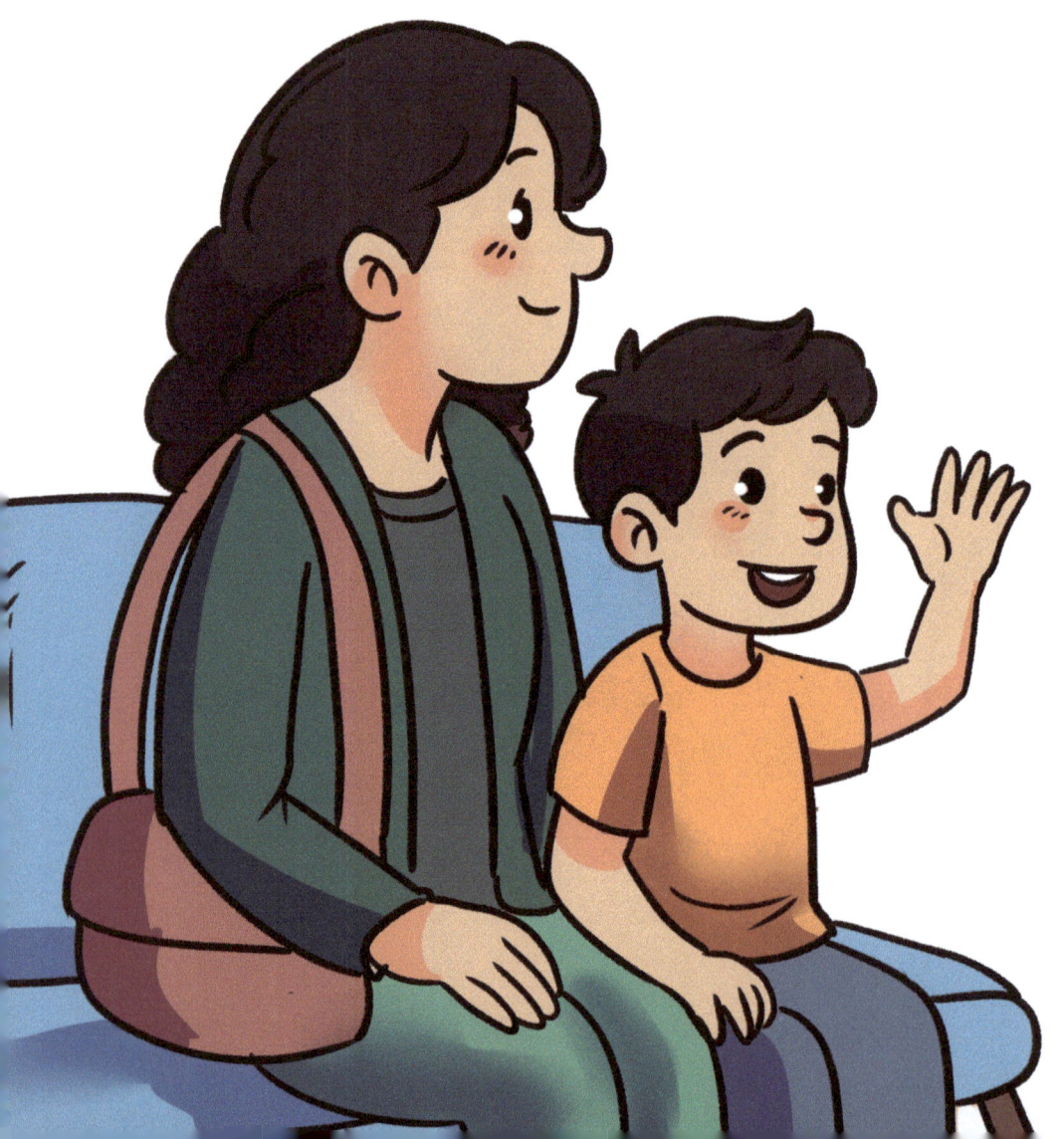

Everyone is here to cheer you on!

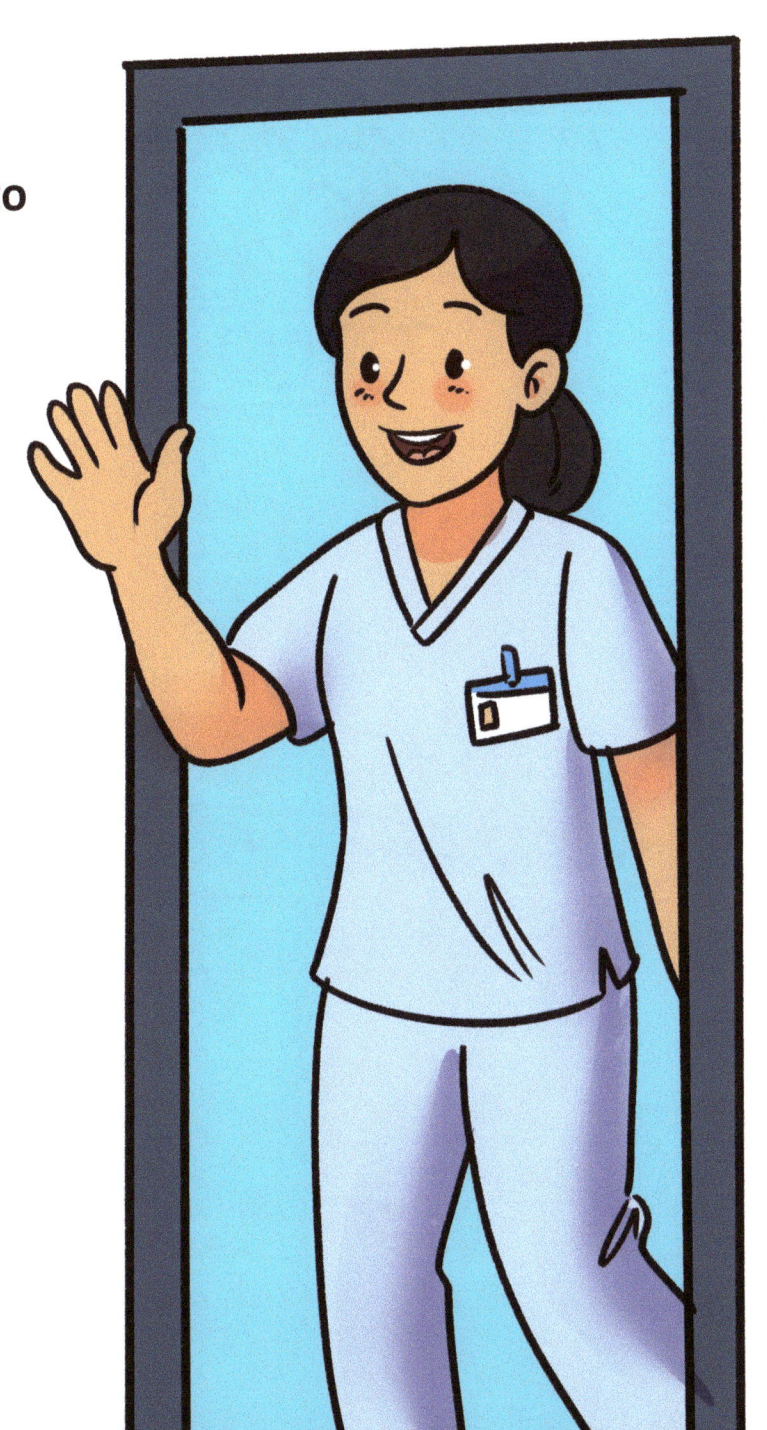

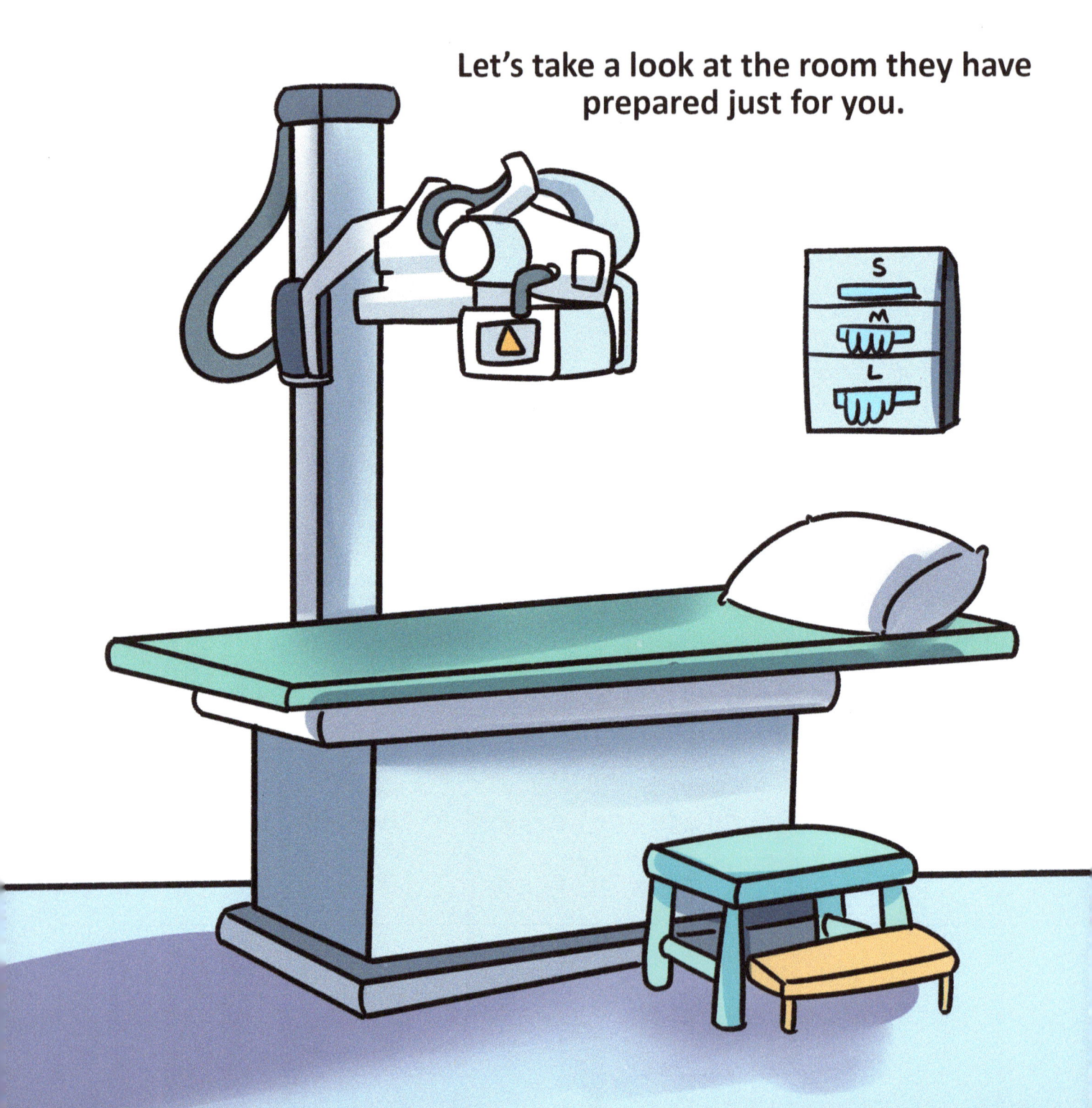

Can you find these things?

- [ ] A friendly staff member
- [ ] Boxes of gloves
- [ ] A step stool
- [ ] A white pillow
- [ ] An X-ray machine
- [ ] A lead apron
- [ ] A lead thyroid (neck) shield

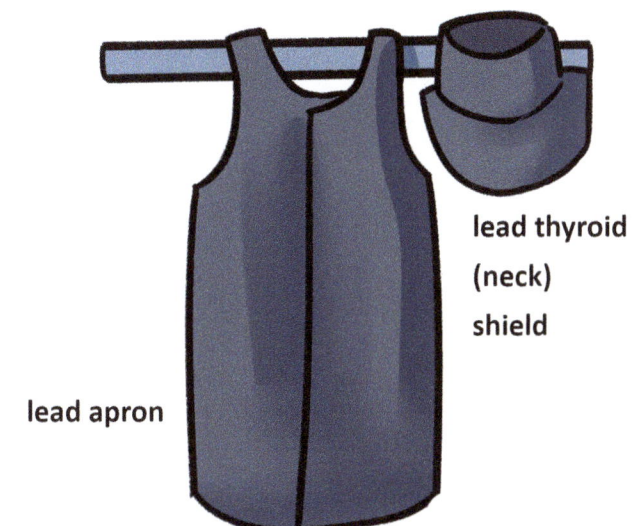

lead apron

lead thyroid (neck) shield

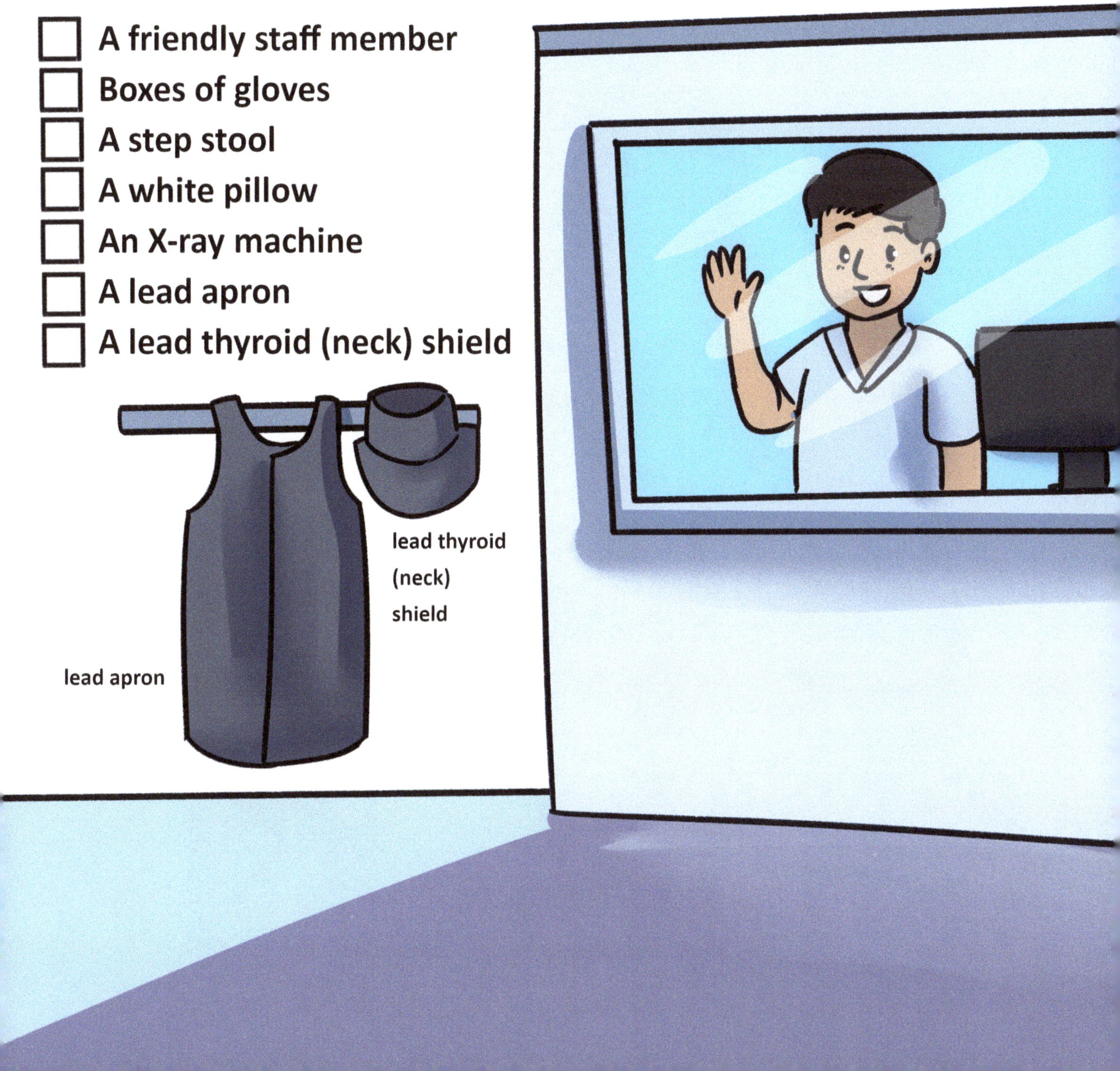

Your X-ray technician will check your wristband and may ask why you need an X-ray. *Can you tell them why you're here?*

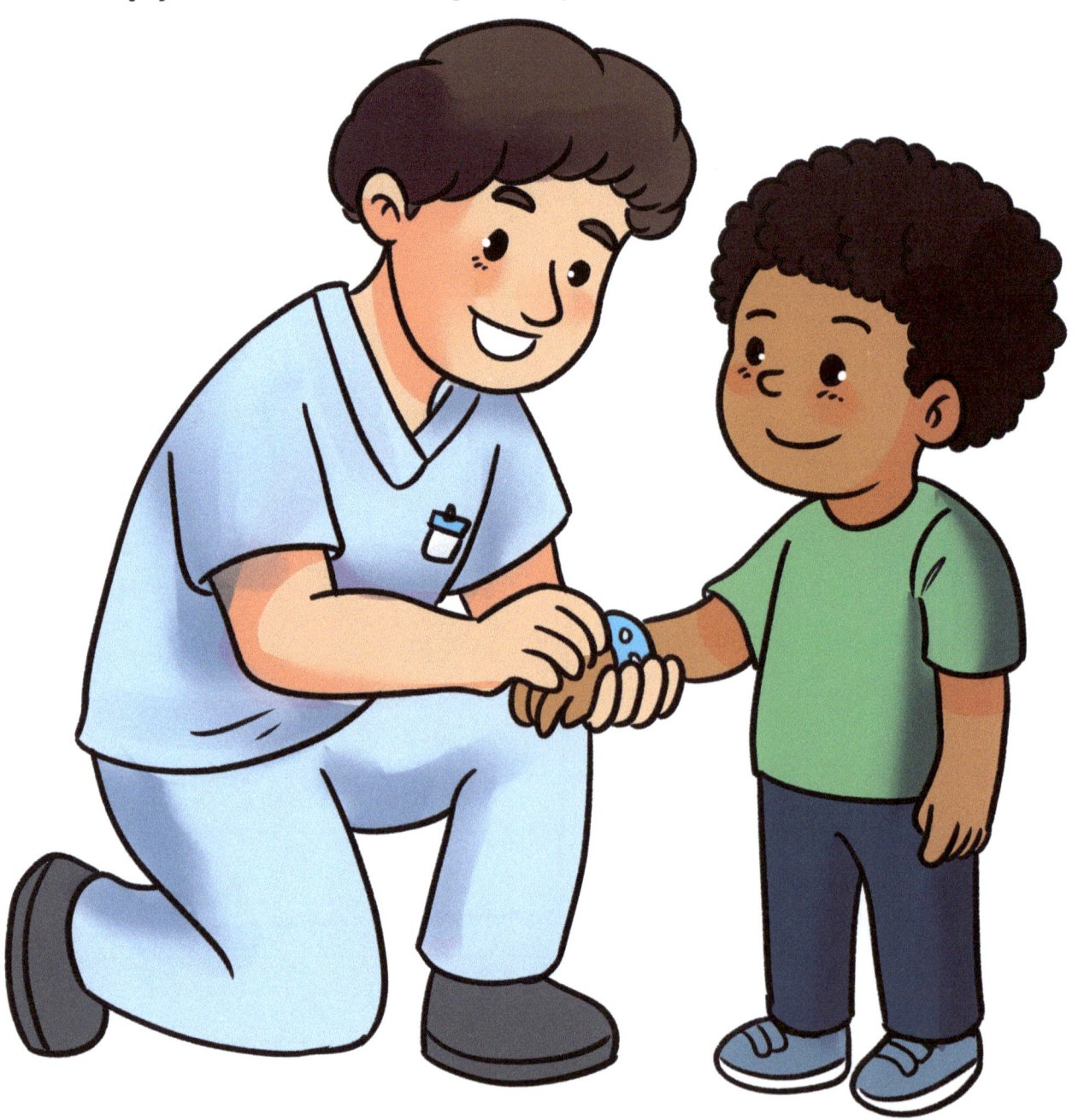

They may also ask where it hurts.
Can you point to the spot?

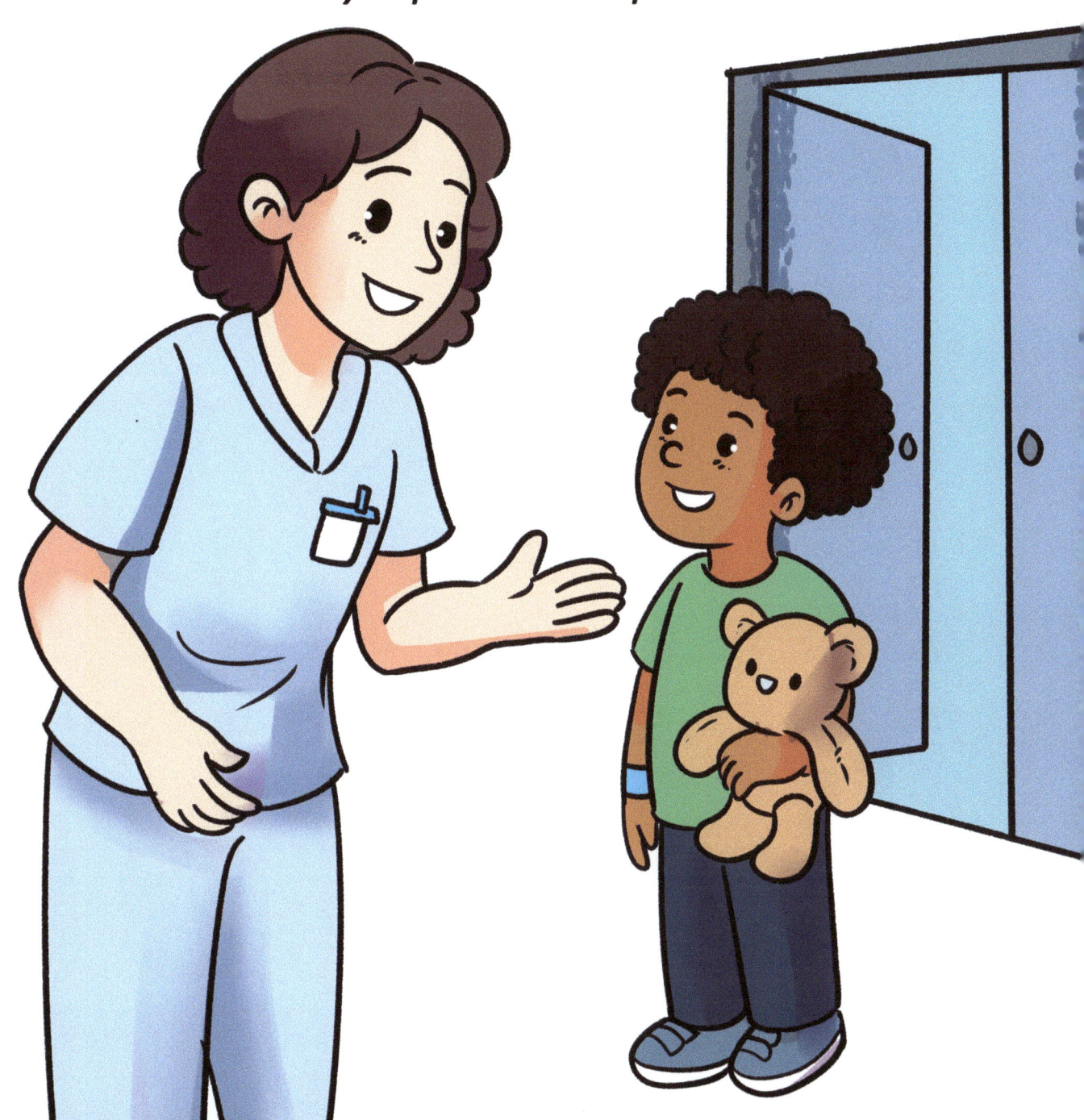

You may need to change into a special gown.
It looks like a superhero cape—but backward!

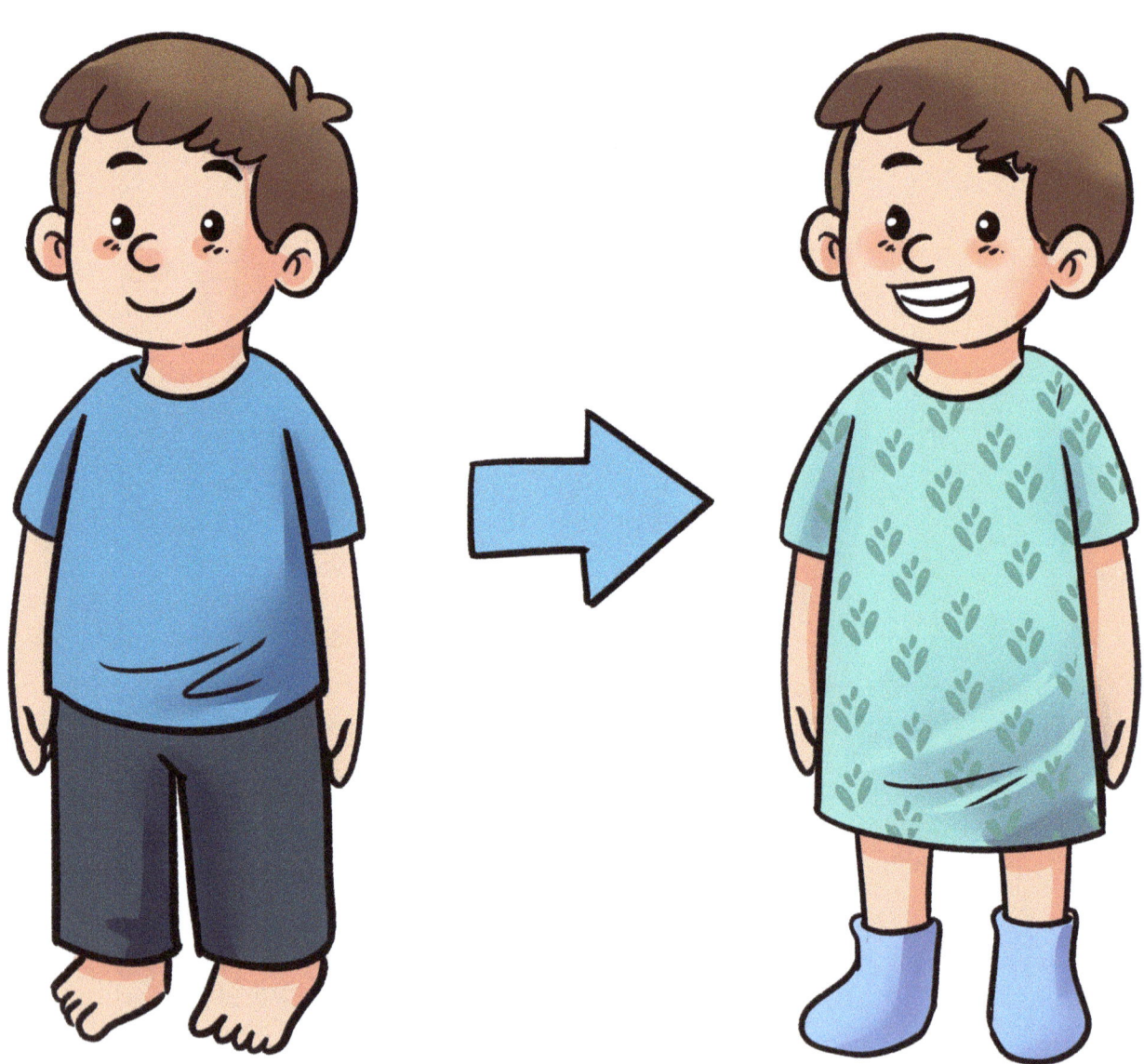

If your parent or guardian stays in the room, they will wear a lead apron to help protect their body.

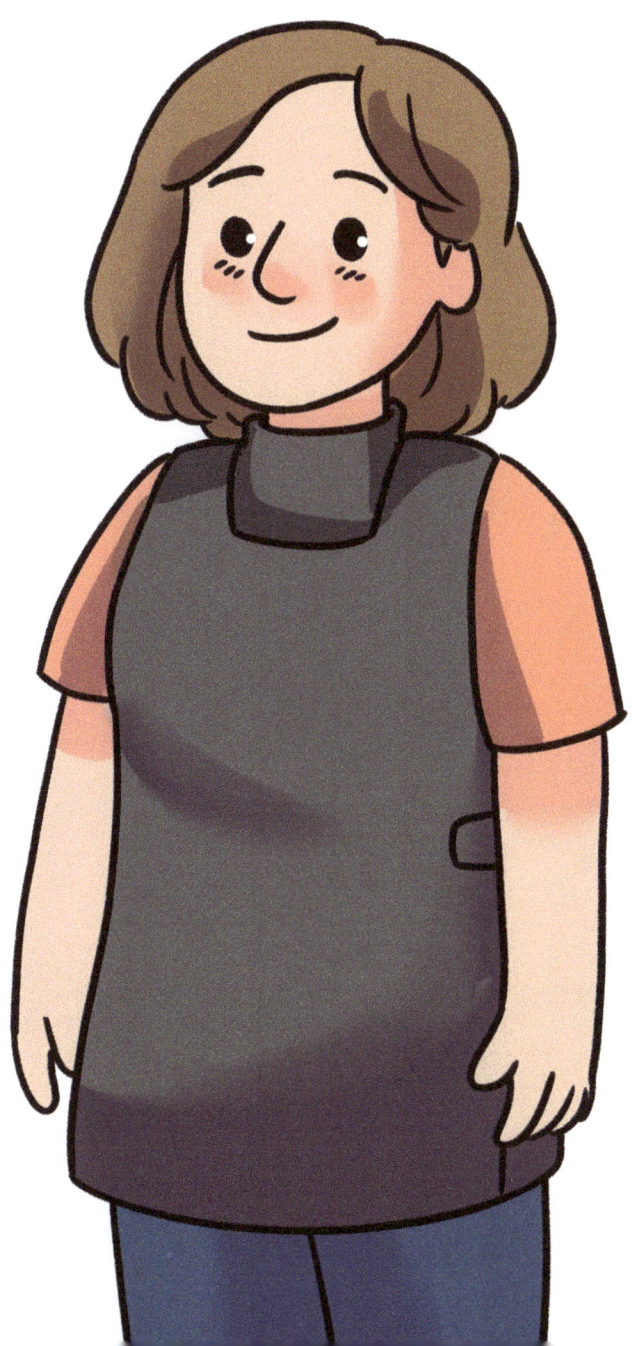

The amount of radiation used for an X-ray picture is very low and does not hurt.

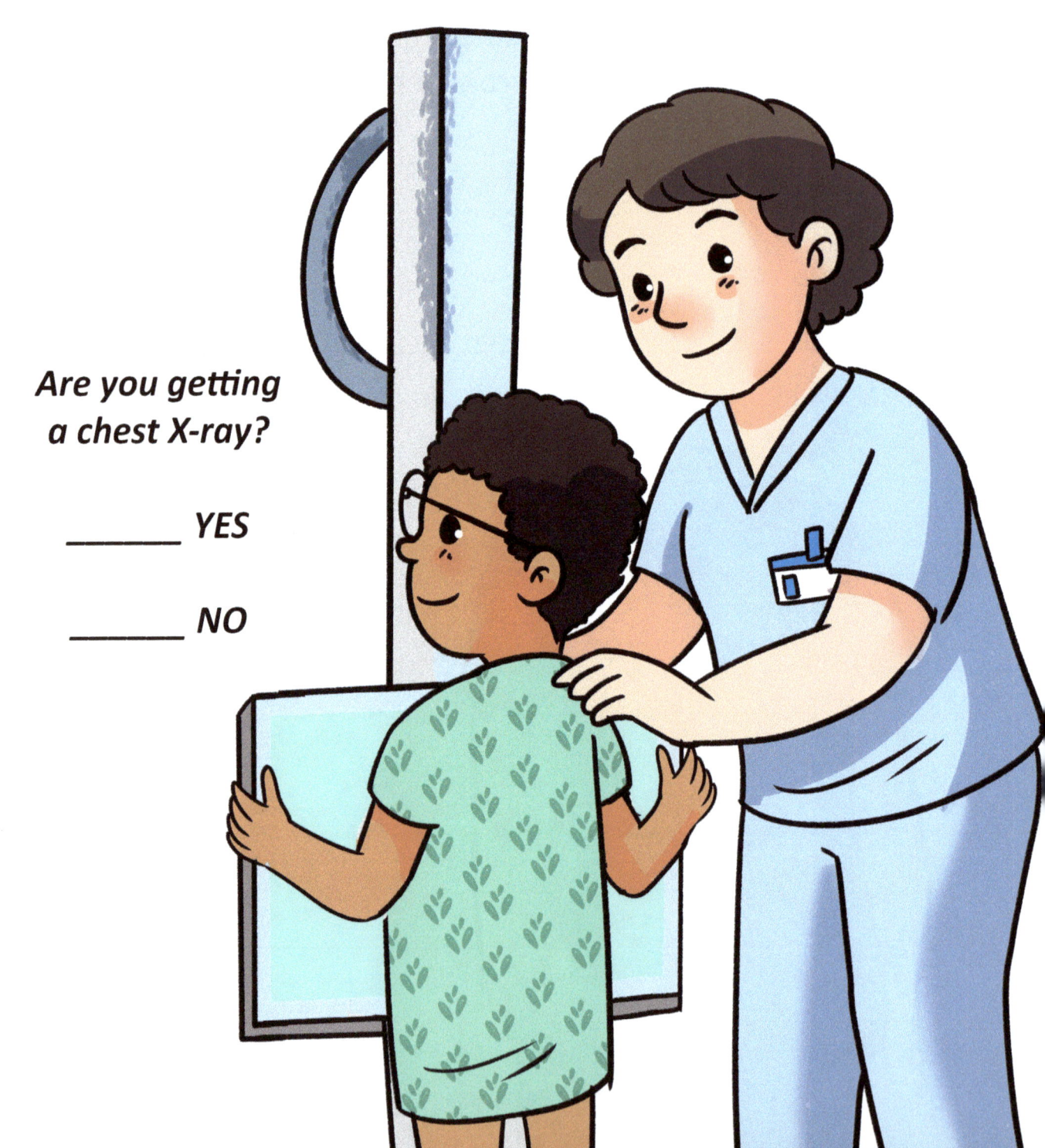

Are you getting a chest X-ray?

_____ YES

_____ NO

Or maybe a finger, hand, wrist, or arm X-ray?

_____ YES   _____ NO

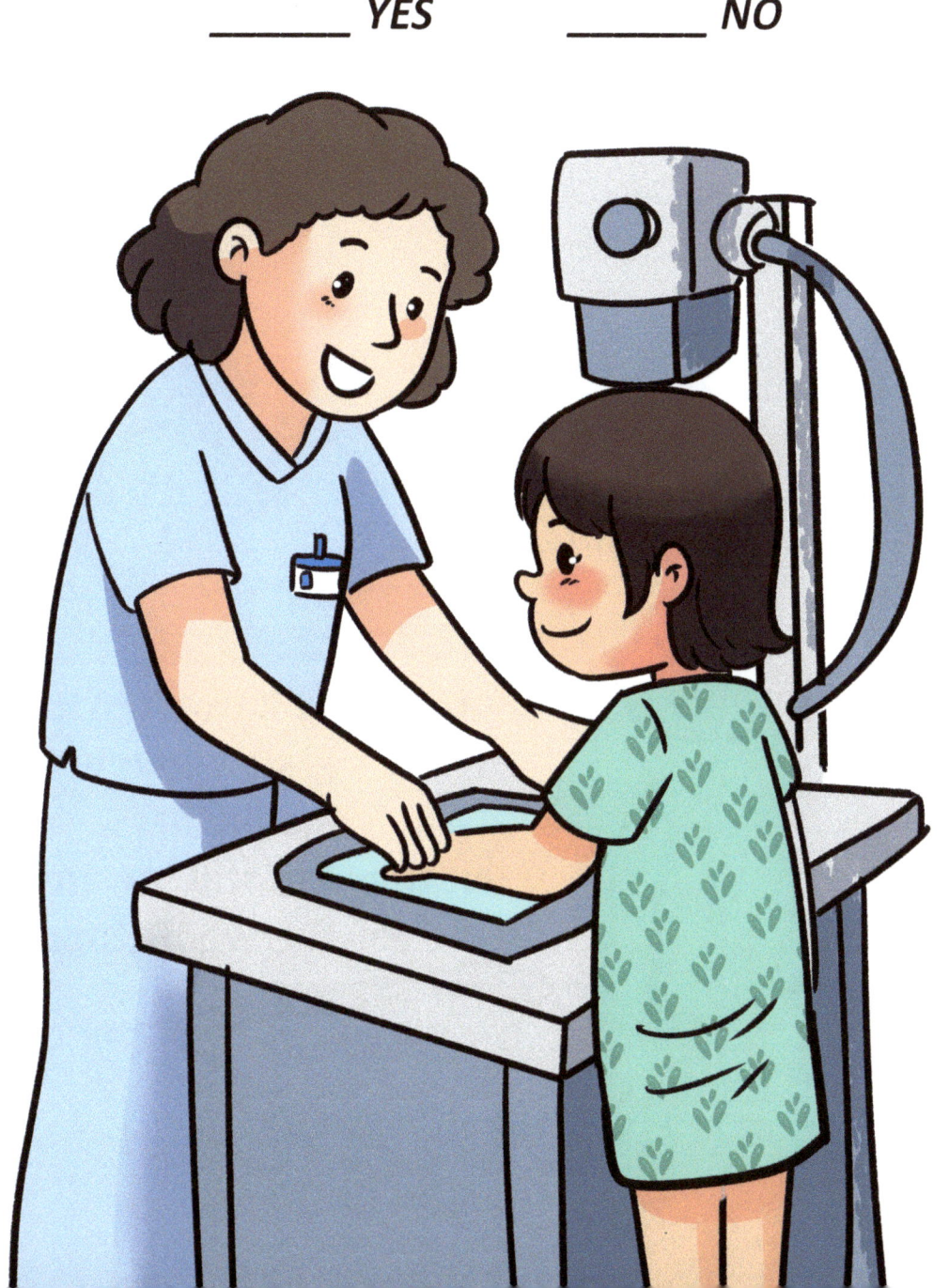

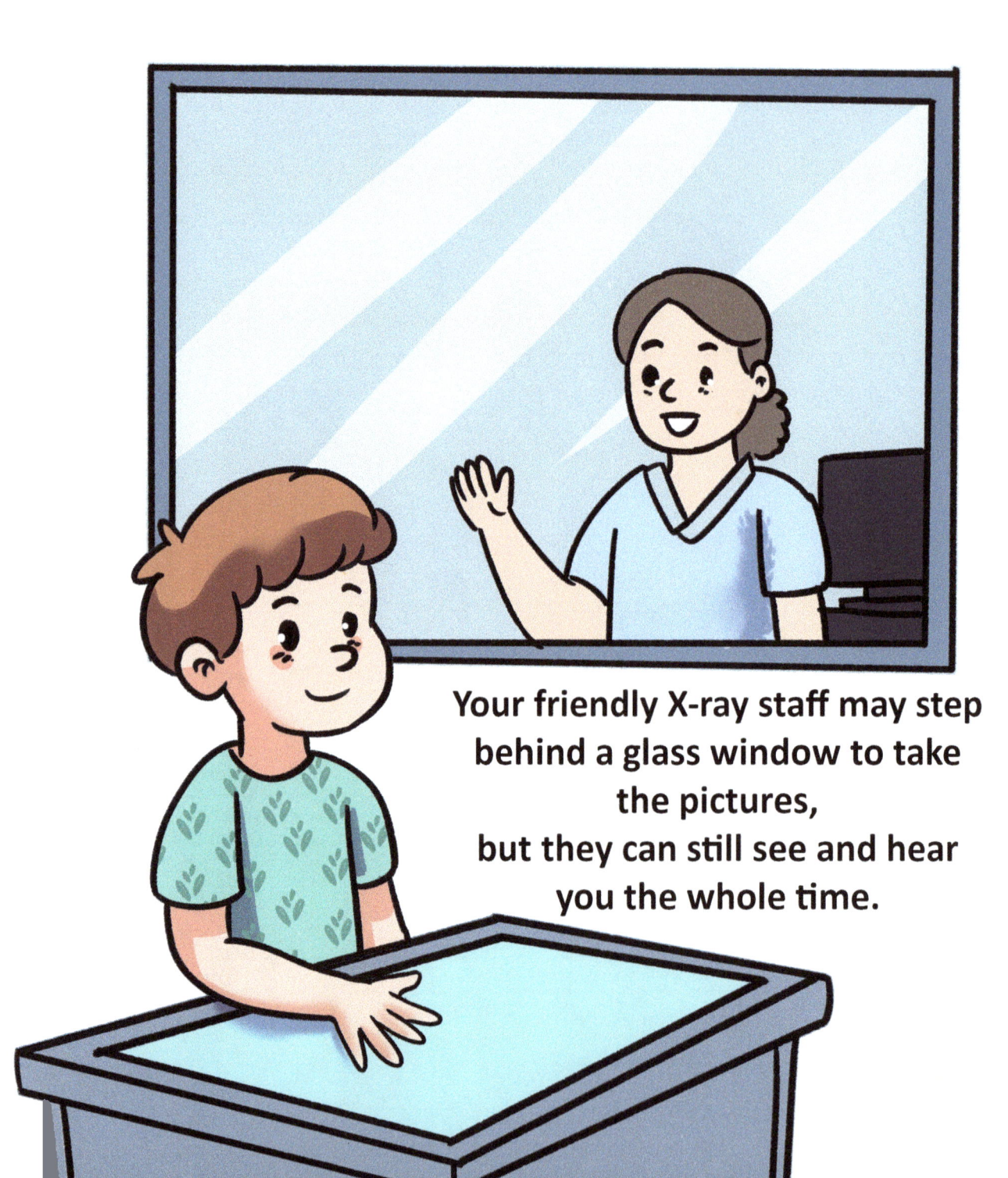

Your friendly X-ray staff may step behind a glass window to take the pictures,
but they can still see and hear you the whole time.

Your grown-up will usually stay close by.

You may or may not need a lead apron—
the staff will let you know.

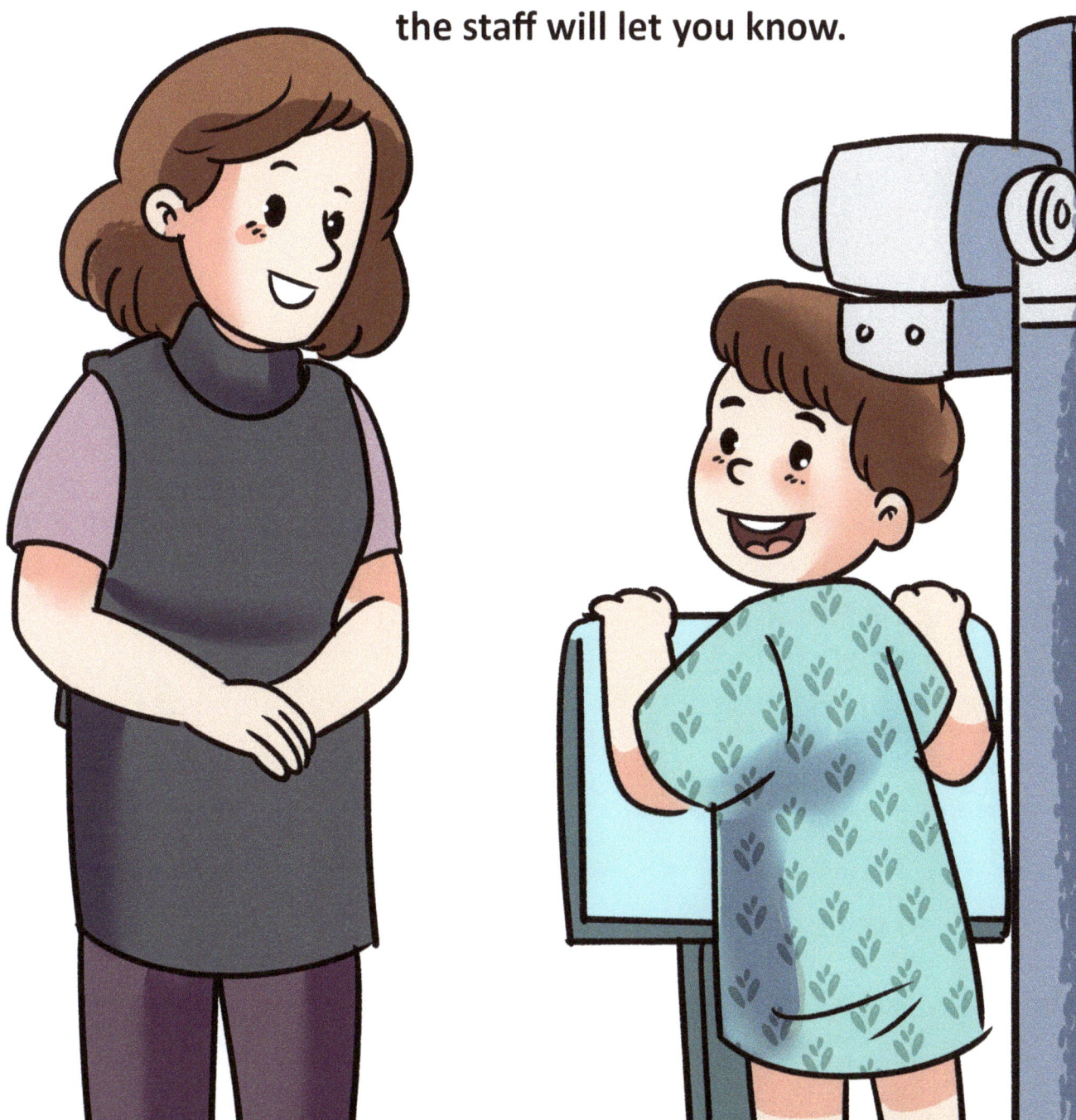

Which X-ray are you getting?

Place a checkmark (✓) next to the one you need.

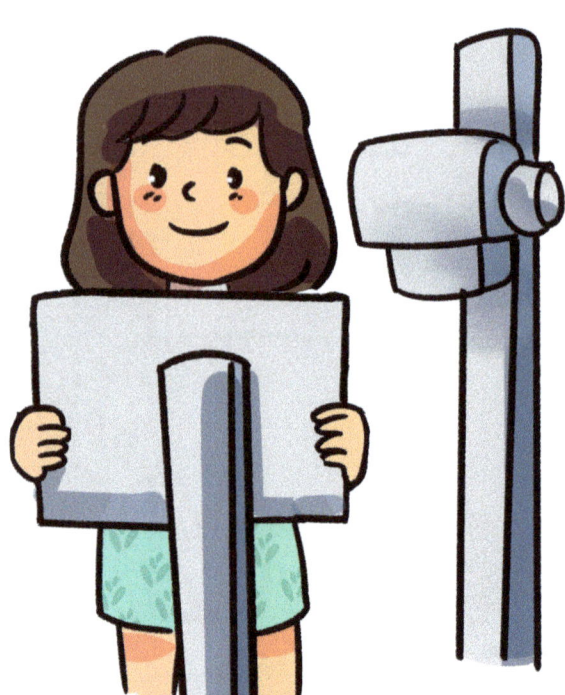

☐ Chest X-ray

Depending on the X-ray, you might be standing, sitting, or lying down.

Swallow study ☐

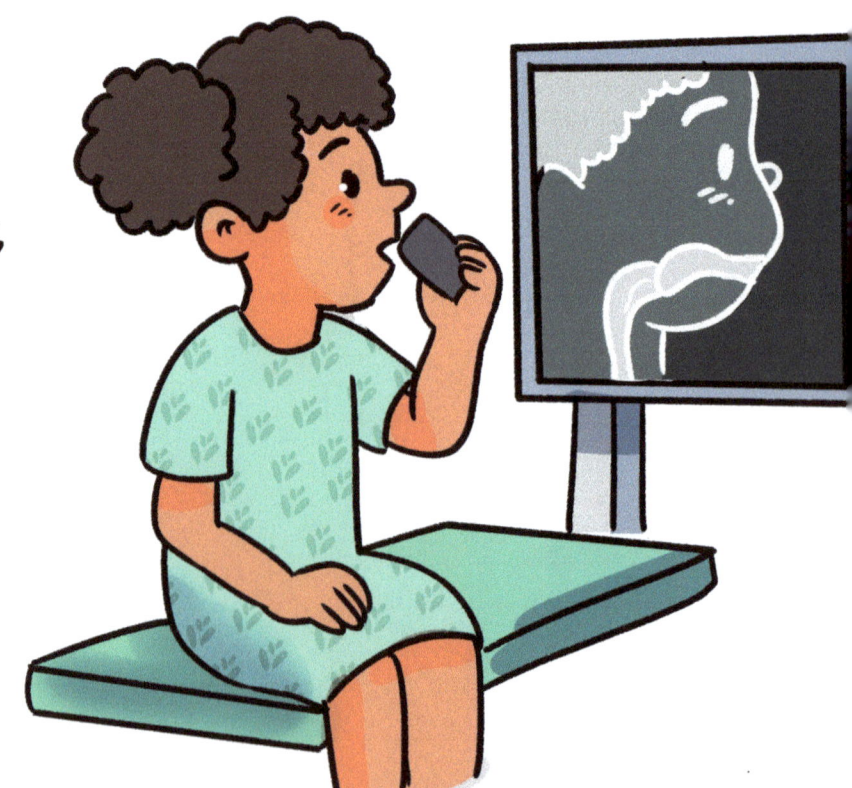

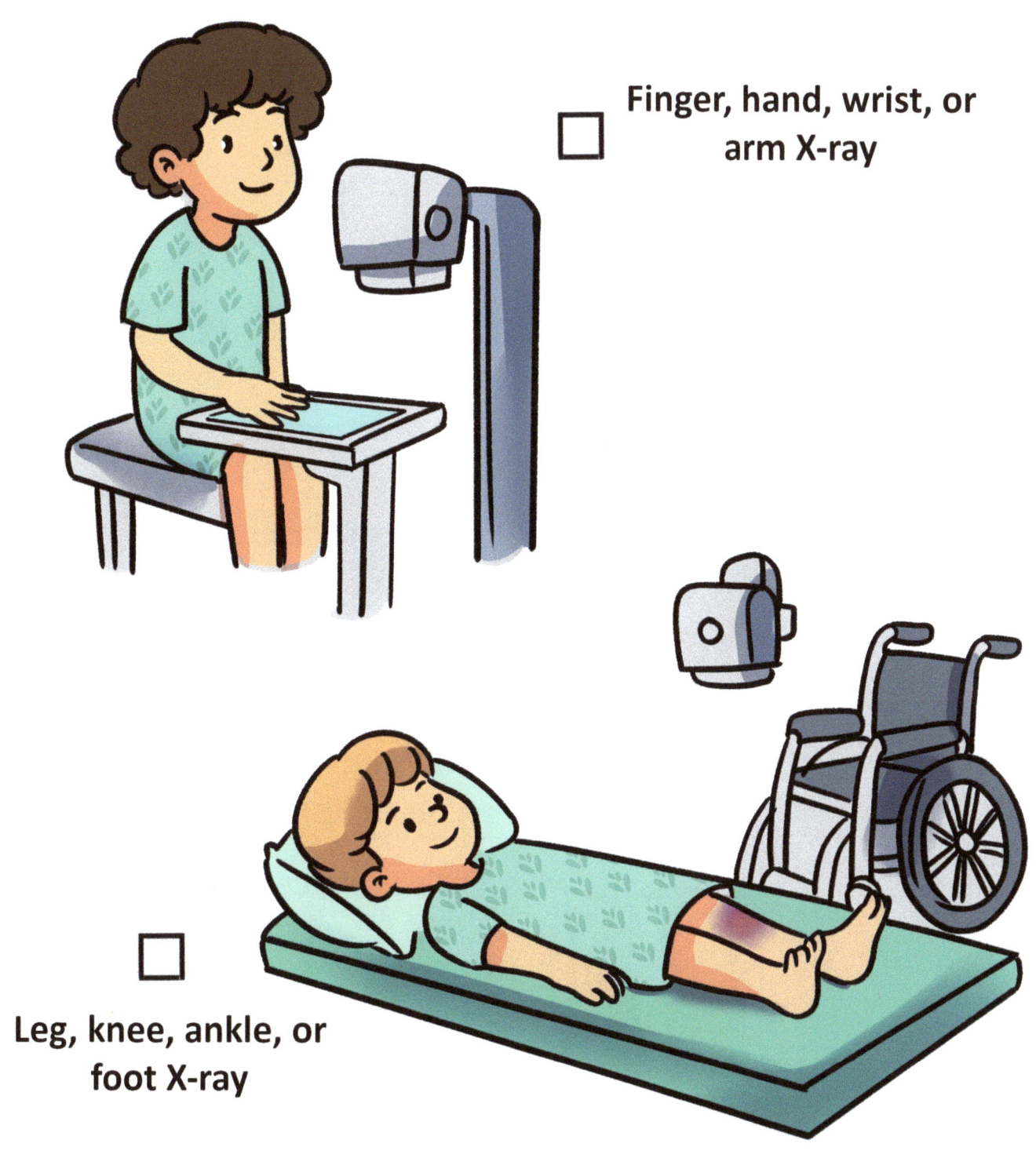

☐ Finger, hand, wrist, or arm X-ray

☐ Leg, knee, ankle, or foot X-ray

Getting an X-ray is quick and doesn't hurt.
If you're getting a chest X-ray,
you'll take a big breath in, hold it, and stay very still.

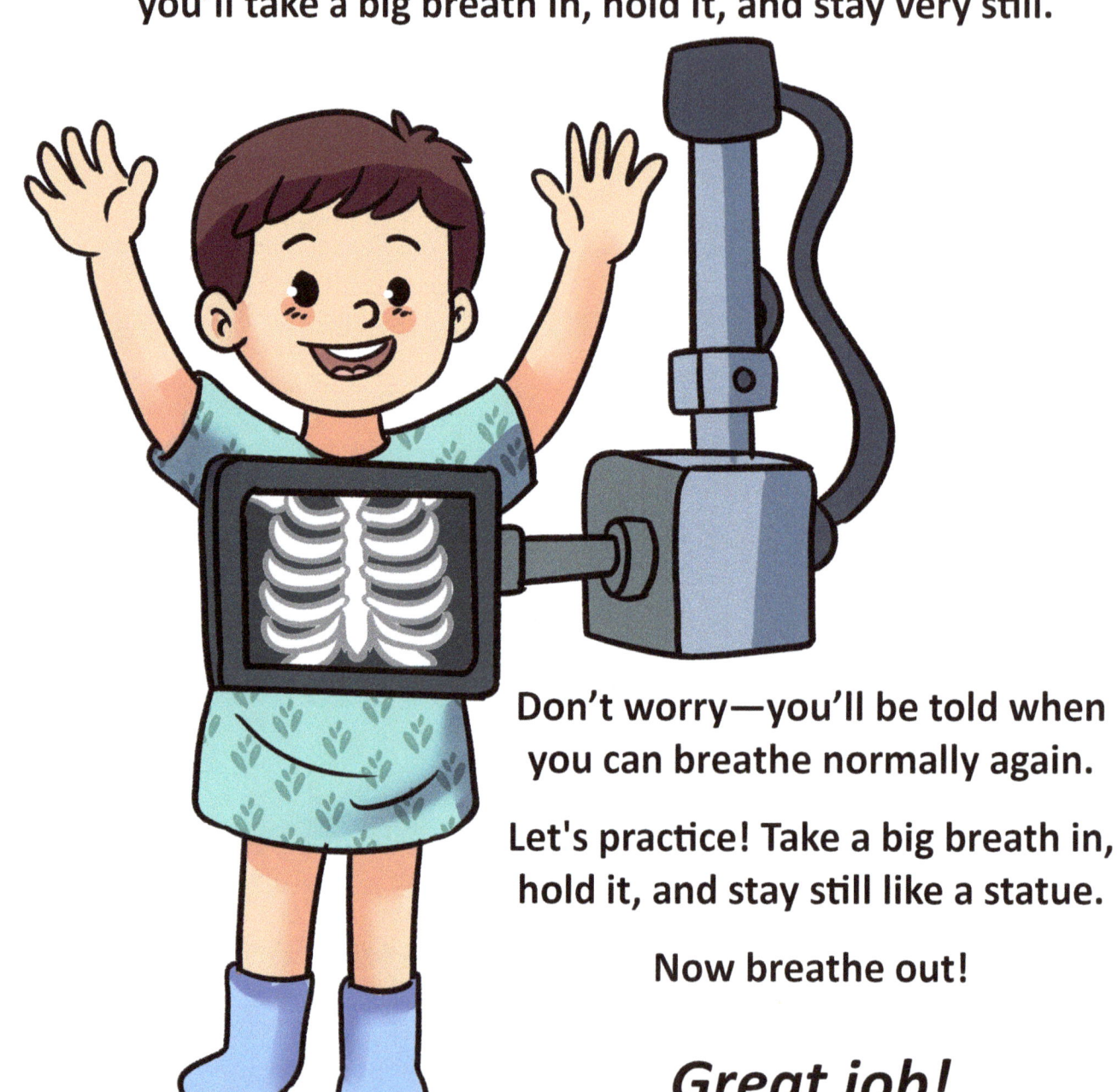

Don't worry—you'll be told when you can breathe normally again.

Let's practice! Take a big breath in, hold it, and stay still like a statue.

Now breathe out!

Great job!

Sometimes, you need to change positions to get different pictures of the same body part.

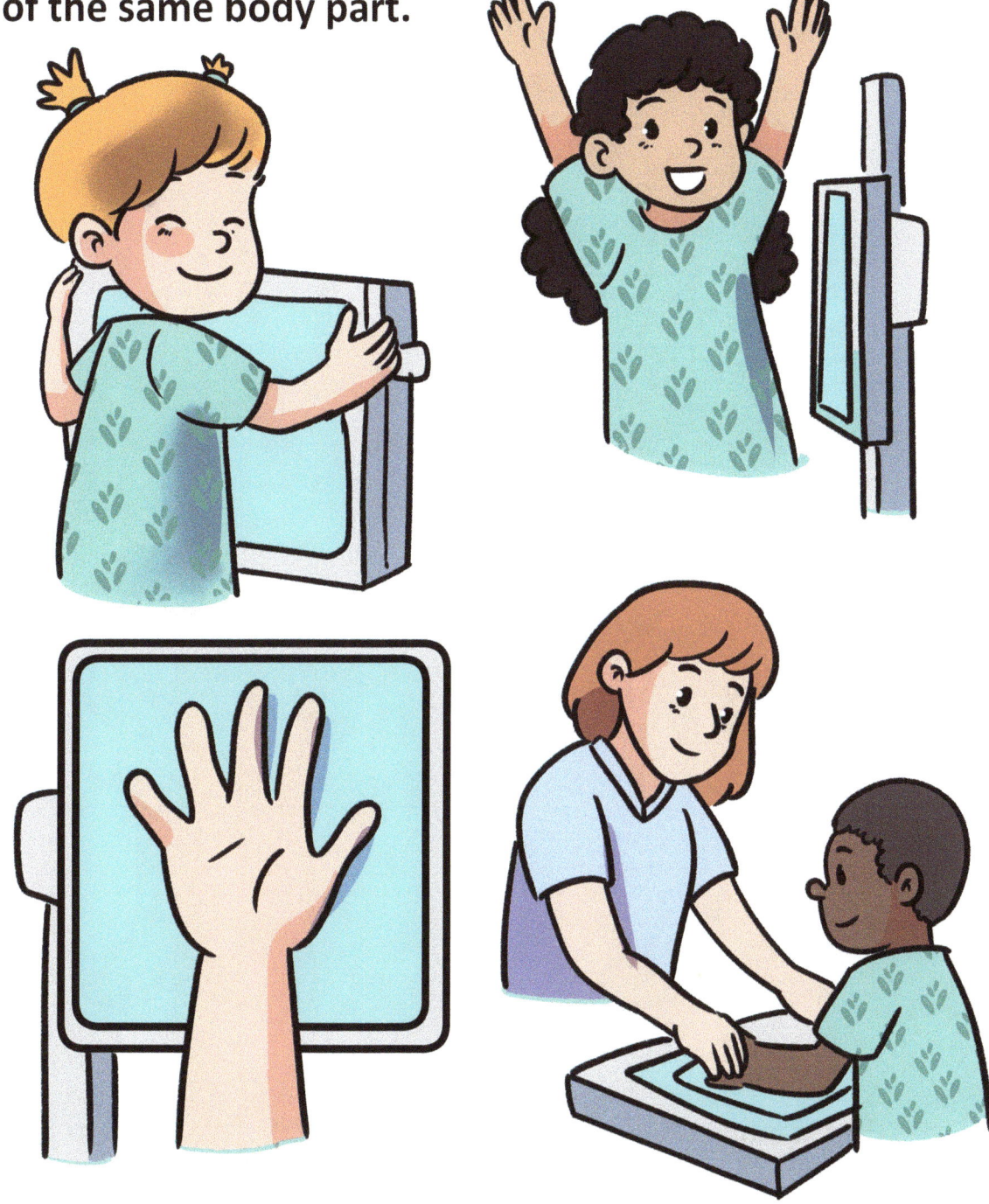

To get clear pictures, it's important to stay very still.

If a picture is blurry, it might need to be taken again— and that's okay.

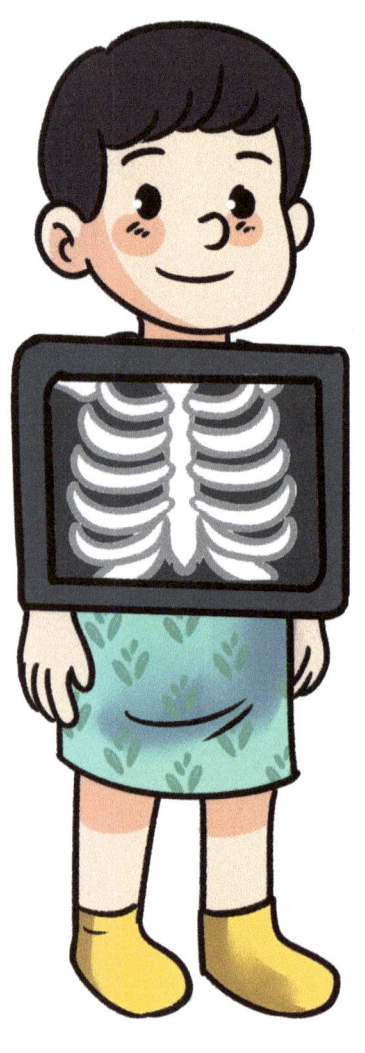

**clear
(staying still)**

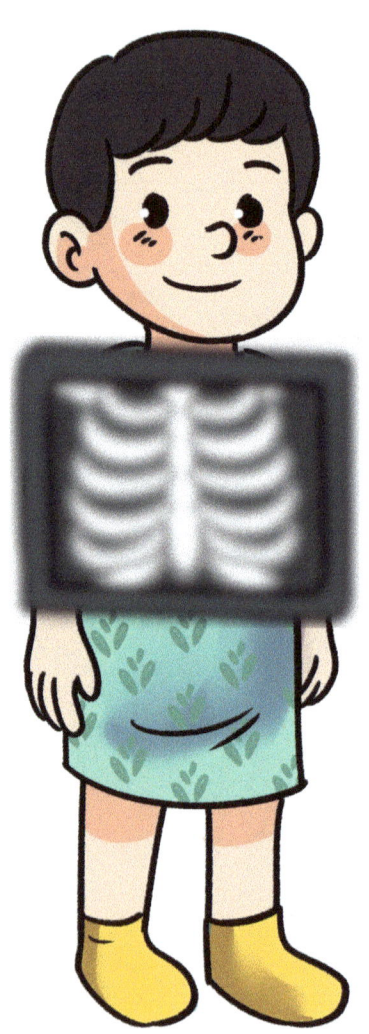

**blurry
(with movement)**

You might wear a lead apron to protect another part of your body.

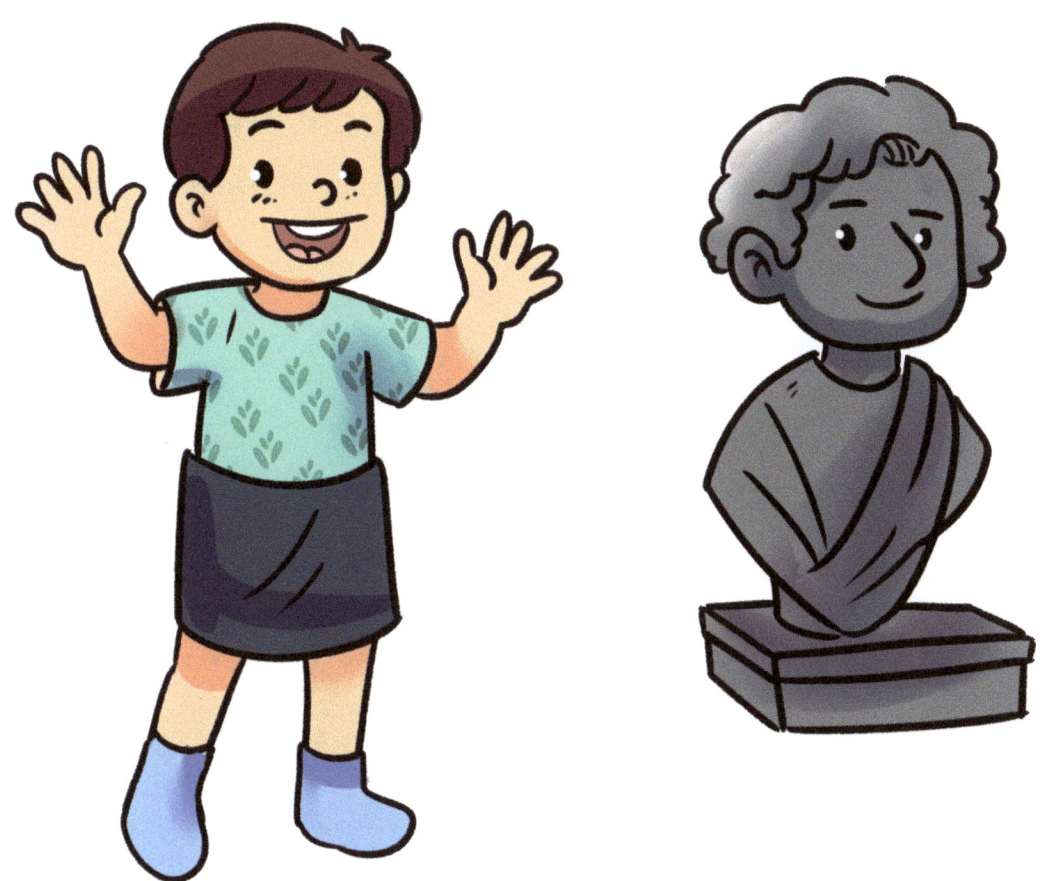

Let's practice staying still,
like playing freeze or pretending to be a statue.

Are you ready?

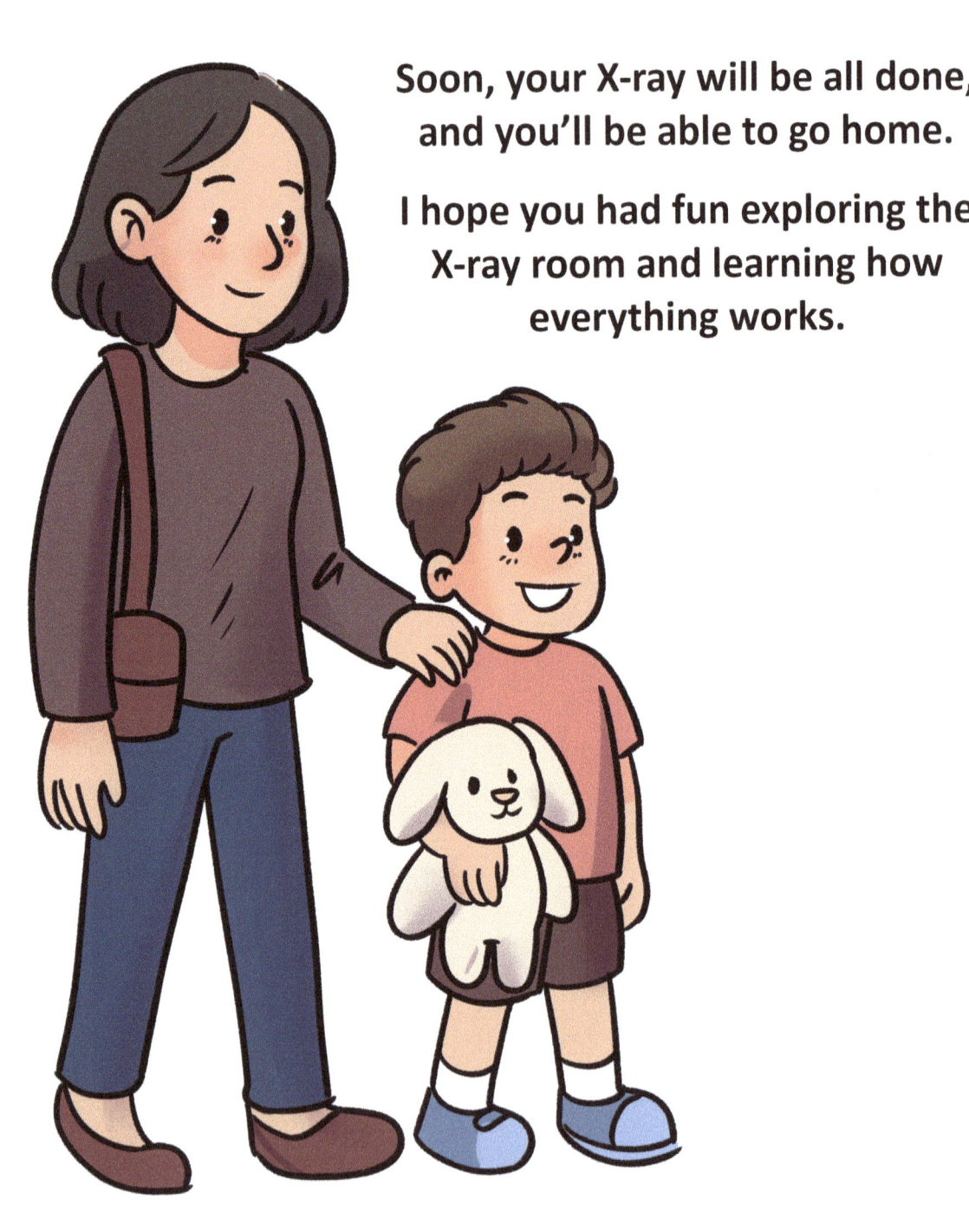

Soon, your X-ray will be all done, and you'll be able to go home.

I hope you had fun exploring the X-ray room and learning how everything works.

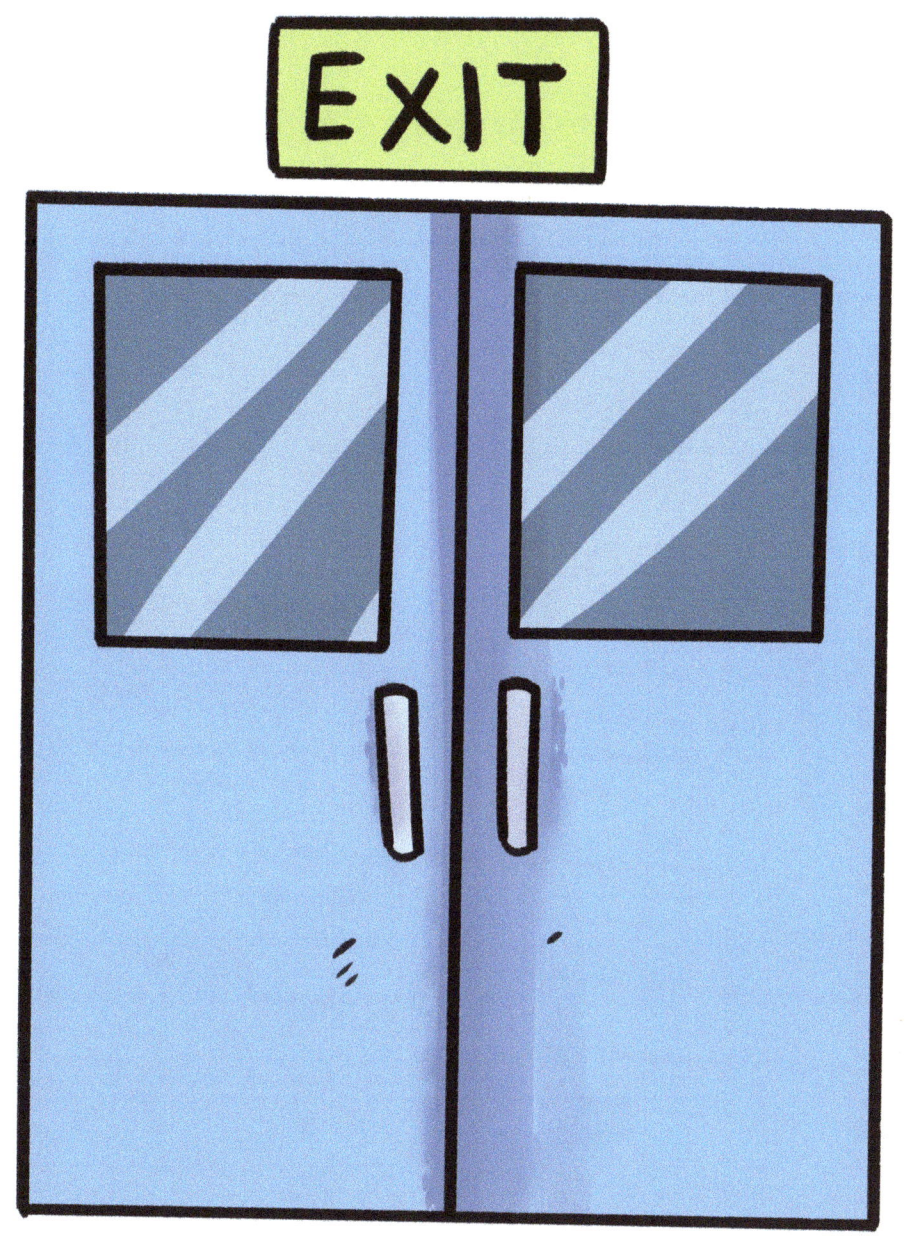

You've been so brave!

Your X-ray pictures will be looked at by doctors who are experts at reading them.

They will send a report to your doctor to help them understand what's happening in your body.

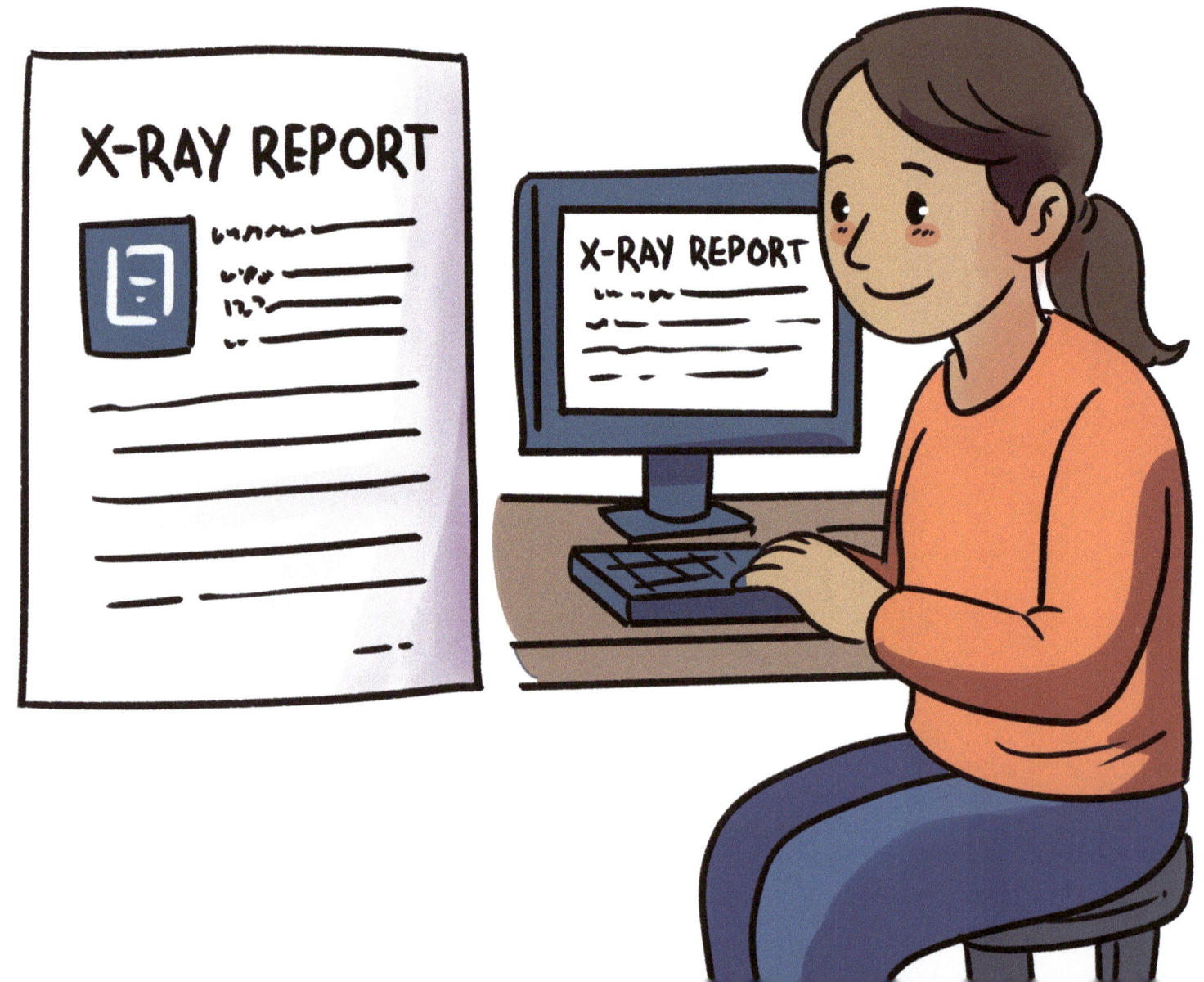

Sometimes your grown-up will get a phone call about the results.

Other times, your doctor will talk to them in person and make a plan to help you feel better.

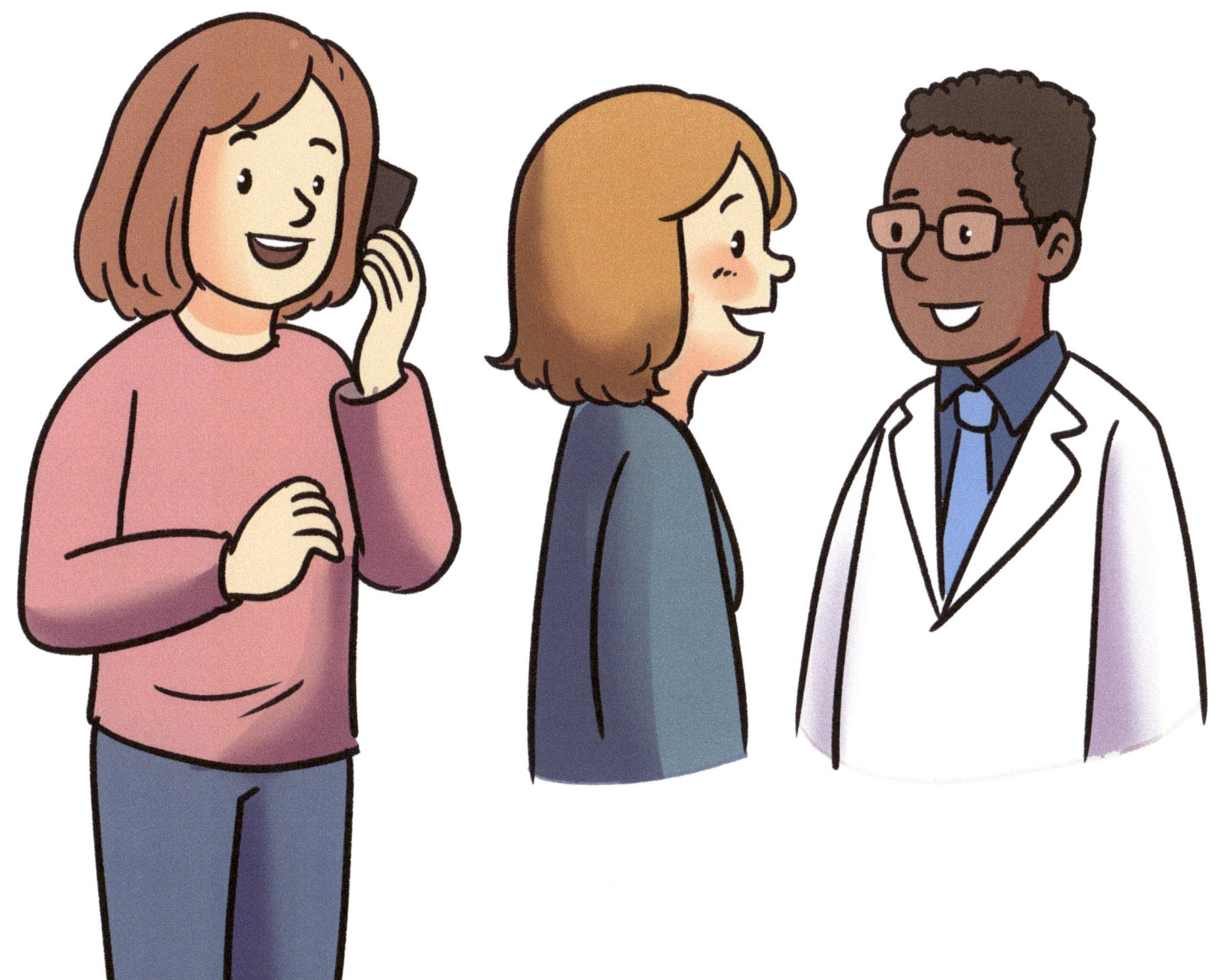

What will you do after your X-ray?

A party? A celebration?

What's your favorite way to celebrate?

Draw or write your party plan below.

Speedy recovery!

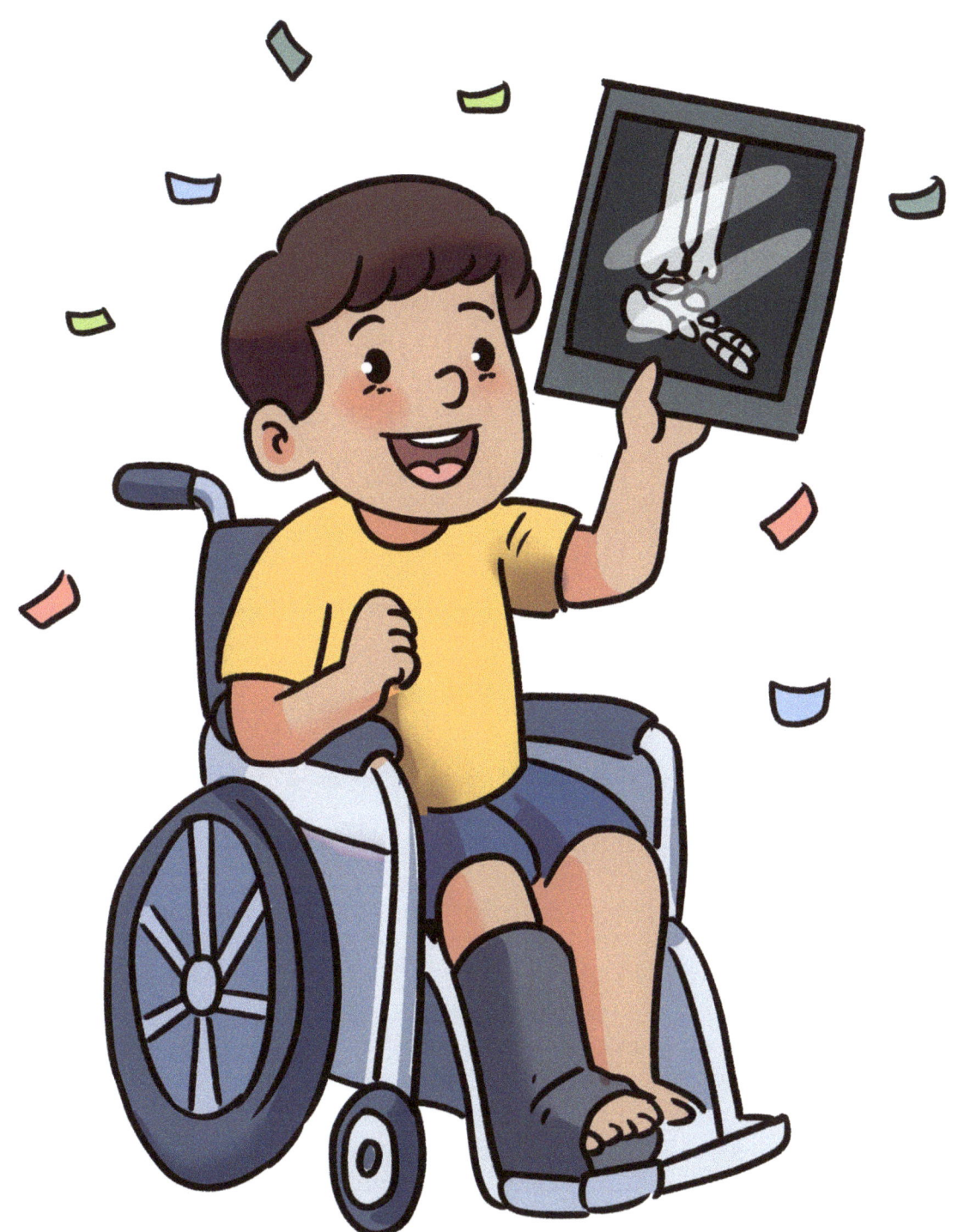

Did this picture book help your child in some way?
If so, I would love to hear about it!

www.amazon.com/gp/product-review/B0GFXW18VX

For other book titles, please visit:

www.fzwbooks.com

Connect with the Author

email: books@fzwbooks.com
facebook/instagram: @FZWbooks

Disclaimer

Please note that the illustrations are not drawn to scale.

This book is written for informational, educational, and personal growth purposes and should not be used as a substitute for medical advice.

Please consult your child's doctor if they need medical attention and to ensure the information in this book pertains to your child's medical condition and needs. I cannot guarantee what your child experiences is exactly what is being discussed in this book.

The author and the publisher are not responsible, either directly or indirectly, for any damages, monetary losses, or reparations due to information in this book. By reading this book, the readers agree not to hold the author and the publisher responsible for any losses as a result of any errors, inaccuracies, or omissions in this book.

Please keep in mind that your child's experience depends on the location, the facility, their medical condition, and the healthcare team. Please use this book in conjunction with your child's doctor's advice. Thank you.

Books by the author

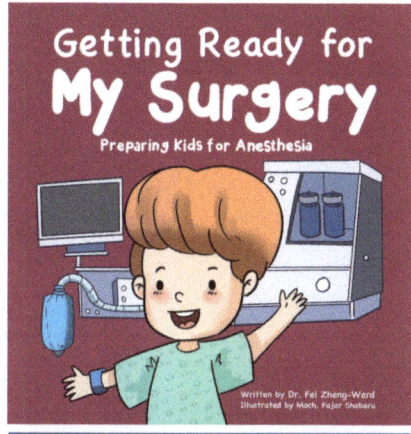 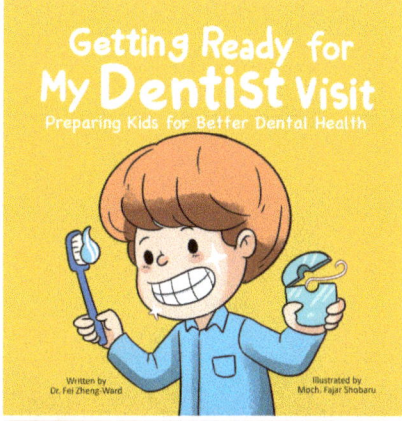 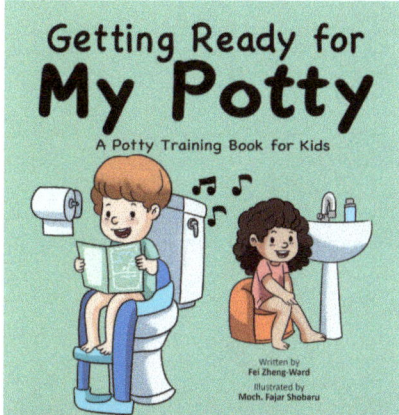
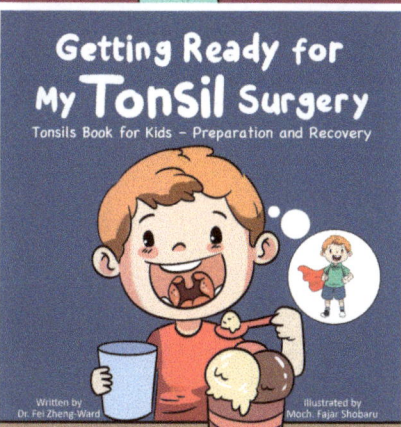 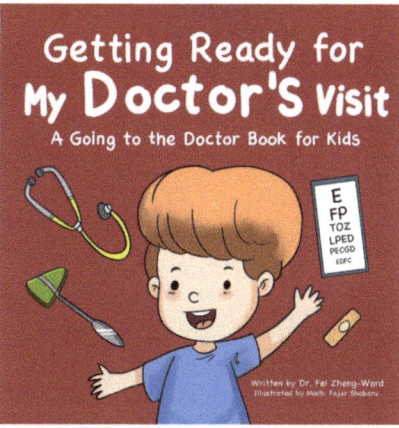 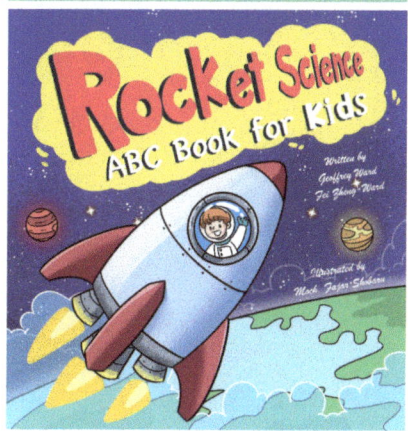
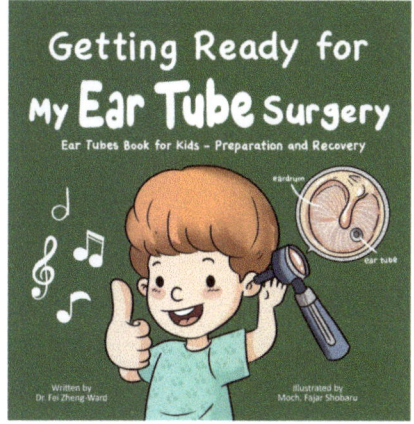 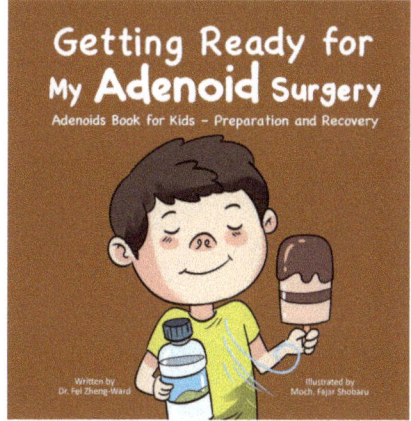 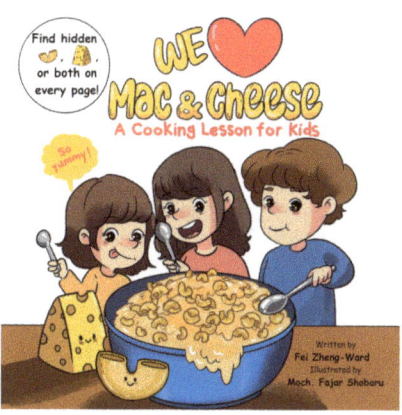

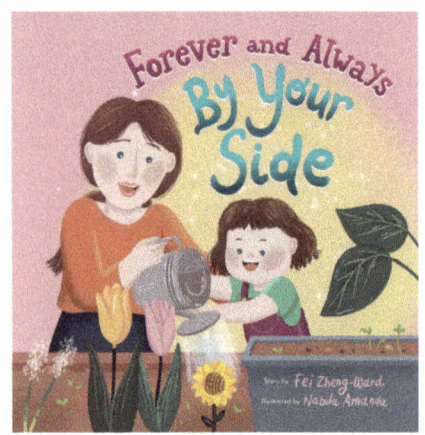
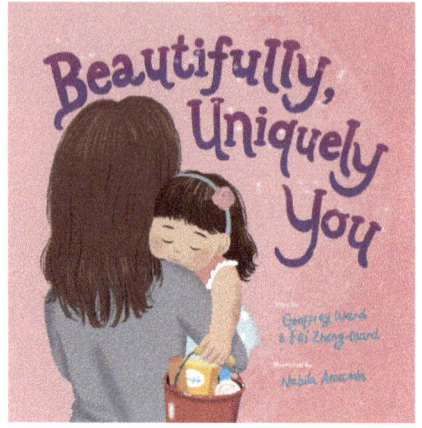
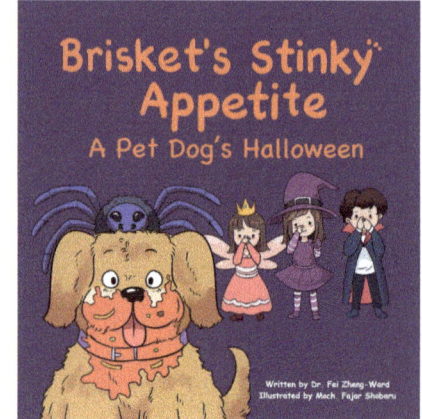
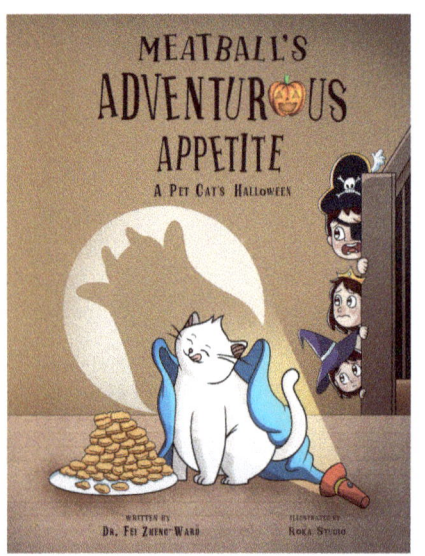
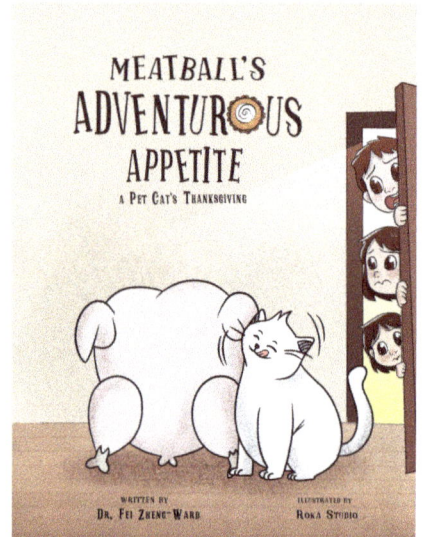
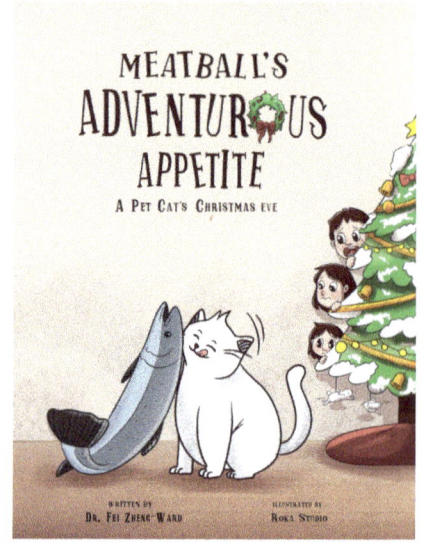
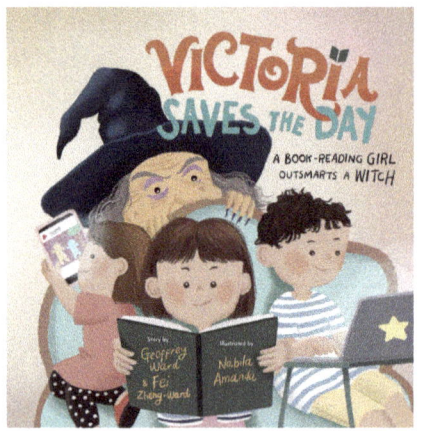
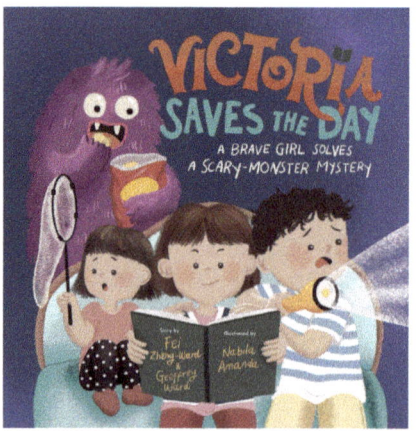
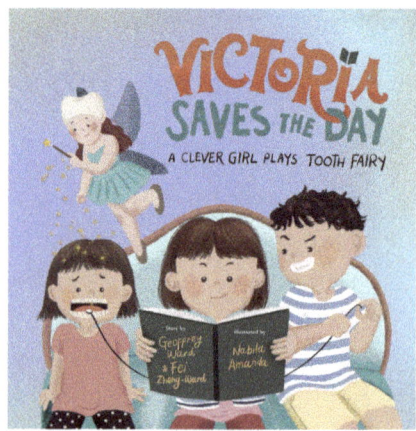

www.ingramcontent.com/pod-product-compliance
Lightning Source LLC
Chambersburg PA
CBHW040000040426
42337CB00032B/5170